医学影像学专业英语

段云燕 孙 静 主编

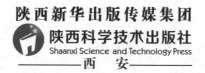

图书在版编目（CIP）数据

  医学影像学专业英语 / 段云燕，孙静主编 . —西安：陕西科学技术出版社，2022.5
  ISBN 978-7-5369-8291-8

  Ⅰ.①医… Ⅱ.①段… ②孙… Ⅲ.①影象诊断 – 英语 – 教材 Ⅳ.① R445

  中国版本图书馆 CIP 数据核字（2021）第 251318 号

医学影像学专业英语
段云燕　孙　静　主编

责任编辑	闫彦敬　付　琨
封面设计	朵云文化

出 版 者	陕西新华出版传媒集团　陕西科学技术出版社
	西安市曲江新区登高路 1388 号陕西新华出版传媒产业大厦 B 座
	电话（029）81205187　传真（029）81205155　邮编 710061
	http://www.snstp.com
发 行 者	陕西新华出版传媒集团　陕西科学技术出版社
	电话（029）81205180　81206809
印　　刷	西安市久盛印务有限责任公司
规　　格	787mm×1092mm　16 开本
印　　张	14.75
字　　数	220 千字
版　　次	2022 年 5 月第 1 版
	2022 年 5 月第 1 次印刷
书　　号	ISBN 978-7-5369-8291-8
定　　价	78.00 元

版权所有　翻印必究

《医学影像学专业英语》编委会

主　　编：段云燕　孙　静
副 主 编：张　璐　李　鹏
编　　者：段云燕（西安医学院）
　　　　　孙　静（西安医学院）
　　　　　张　璐（商洛市中心医院）
　　　　　李　鹏（青岛滨海学院附属医院）
　　　　　李金霞（西安医学院）
　　　　　杨　旭（西安医学院）
　　　　　赵宏波（西安医学院）
　　　　　冯　楠（西安医学院）
　　　　　白　燕（西安医学院）
　　　　　纪　超（西安医学院）
　　　　　肖　丹（西安医学院）

目　　录

第一部分　医学英语
第一章　医学英语术语学……………………………………………………… 1
第二章　各系统术语…………………………………………………………… 27
第三章　医院相关英语词汇…………………………………………………… 88

第二部分　医学影像学基础
第一章　医学影像学发展简史………………………………………………… 113
第二章　医学影像设备………………………………………………………… 134
第三章　医学影像检查技术…………………………………………………… 147

第三部分　医学影像诊断病例及影像报告
第一章　医学影像诊断病例…………………………………………………… 162
第二章　医学影像诊断报告…………………………………………………… 183

附录　国外影像医学临床与教学…………………………………………… 203

参考文献……………………………………………………………………… 228

第一部分　医学英语

第一章　医学英语术语学

一、英语及医学英语发展简史

英语属于应用非常广泛的印欧语系，它包括目前大多数的欧洲语言。尽管缺乏相应的书面记录，但原始印欧语系对英语的影响至今可见。比如，父亲"father"这个词在德语中为"vater"，希腊语为"pater"，波斯语为"pedar"，拉丁语为"pater"，梵语为"pitr"。这些词都通过共同的同源，即同源词来互相联系。

在印欧语系的所有分支中，有两个最为重要的语系，即日耳曼语系和罗曼语系。

（一）古英语（450年—1100年）

在五六世纪，来自德国北部、丹麦和荷兰北部的盎格鲁人、撒克逊人和朱特人入侵了不列颠群岛，并开始在这些地区定居。这些入侵者被称之为盎格鲁－撒克逊人，他们将最初会讲凯尔特语的居民从现在的英格兰、威尔士、康沃尔郡和爱尔兰赶出，并留下了一些凯尔特语言。他们说盎格鲁撒克逊语，可以相互理解，并在某种程度上发展成我们所说的古英语。现代英语中约有一半最常用的单词来源于古英语词根。例如，water, stone, foot, fire, sheep 和 strong 都源于古英语词根。

（二）诺曼征服与中古英语（1100—1500年）

征服者威廉，诺曼底公爵，威廉一世国王于1066年入侵并征服了英格兰和盎格鲁-撒克逊人。新的征服者讲述的是法语方言，称为盎格鲁-诺曼语。诺曼人也是日耳曼语种，盎格鲁-诺曼人是法国方言，除了基本的拉丁语根源外，还具有相当大的日耳曼语影响力。

在诺曼征服之前，拉丁语对英语的影响很小，但现在大量输入了罗曼史（盎格鲁-诺曼）一词。诺曼人的影响力几乎遍及各个领域，从政府、法律领域到艺术和文学领域，都可以通过两个词来说明："牛肉"和"牛"。"牛肉"通常由贵族食用，起源于盎格鲁-诺曼底人，而养牛的盎格鲁-撒克逊人则保留了日耳曼"牛"。许多法律术语，例如起诉书，陪审团和判决书都起源于盎格鲁-诺曼底，因为诺曼底人是由法院管理的。这种分裂在许多情况下都可以看到，在这种情况下，贵族通常使用的词具有浪漫的根源，而盎格鲁-撒克逊人的常用术语则具有日耳曼语的根源。从法语中借用的其他词包括 pork, govern, administer, beauty, music, painting, colour, champagne, fashion 等。两种语言的混合被称为中古英语。中古英语最著名的例子是乔叟的坎特伯雷故事集。与古英语不同，尽管有些阅读起来困难，但现代英语使用者可以阅读中古英语。

14世纪后期，人们开始了在官方场合恢复英语的使用。1356年，伦敦市长和议员要求使用英语进行法庭诉讼。1362年，大臣首次以英语发表演讲，向国会致开幕词。到1362年，贵族和平民之间的语言划分已基本结束。《恳求规约》的通过使英语成为法院的语言，并开始在议会中使用。随着现代英语的兴起，中古英语时代结束于1500年左右。

（三）早期现代英语（1500—1800年）

英语的创新浪潮出现在文艺复兴时期。古典学术的复兴使许多经典的拉丁语和希腊语单词进入英语语言体系。早期现代英语吸纳了希腊的语法，并吸纳了其在逻辑、算术、几何学、天文学和音乐等方面的单词。在此期间，用英语写作最出名的便是威廉·莎士比亚。许多单词和短语是由莎士比亚创造或首次使用的。

（四）晚期现代英语（1800年—现代）

早期现代英语和晚期现代英语之间的主要区别是词汇。它们的发音、语法和拼写方面基本相同，但"晚期现代英语"单词更多。这主要是由两个历史因素造成的。首先是工业革命和技术社会的兴起需要用新词来表达以前不存在的事物和思想。其次是大英帝国的崛起。在鼎盛时期，英国统治着全球的 1/4 领土，英语吸纳了许多外来词并将其变成英语的外来词。

工业和科学革命产生了对新词的需求，用以描述新的创造和发现。为此，英语严重依赖拉丁语和希腊语。Oxygen, protein, nuclear, 和 vaccine 等词在古典语言中并不存在，但它们却源自拉丁语和希腊语。这种新词并非仅源于古典根源。英文词根用于诸如 horsepower, airplane 和 typewriter 之类的术语。今天，这种流行语仍在继续，可以说在电子和计算机领域最为明显。Byte，cyber-，bios，hard-drive 和 microchip 就是很好的例子。

此外，大英帝国的崛起和全球贸易的增长不仅为世界引入了英语，还为英语引入了单词。印地语和印度语系的其他语言为英语发展也提供了许多单词，例如 pundit, shampoo, pajamas 和 juggernaut。实际上，世界上每种语言都为英语的发展做出了贡献，比如芬兰语、日语、法语和拉丁语都做出了巨大贡献。

最后，20 世纪发生的两次世界大战影响了军事英语用语表达，但除了航海用语外，其很少影响标准英语。然而，在 20 世纪中叶，军事用语以前所未有的方式影响了标准英语。比如：blockbuster, nose dive, camouflage, radar, roadblock, spearhead 和 landing strip 都曾是军事术语，已成为标准英语。

二、医学术语的词源研究

医学术语根据其来源，可以分为两大类，即本地术语和借用术语。本地术语是源自古英语的单词，借用术语则是因为它们取自其他语言。除了一小部分源自古英语的医学词汇外，医学术语主要以希腊语、拉丁语和法语词汇为基础，其中希腊语和拉丁语是医学术语中生产力最高的。德语、意大利语、西班牙语和其他语言也为医学术语做出了一些贡献。

（一）古英语演变而来的单词

古英语基本上是从盎格鲁-撒克逊人说的方言发展而来的。古英语中的大多数医学用词表示器官、物质和人类活动的基本概念。在他们的发展过程中，或多或少地发生了变化，涉及语音、形态和语义的变化。

解剖词

ankle：在古英语中，它是 oncleow。人们认为现代形式是从基础 ank-"弯曲"衍生而来的。

back：在古英语中，它是 boec，意思是"向后"。

blood：在古英语中，拼写为 blod，它最初的意思是"肿胀，涌出，喷出"或"爆发的东西"。

chest：在古英语中，其对应的拼写是 cest，意思是"盒子，保险箱"。在 1530 年，这个含义扩展到了"thorax"，取代了 breast。

ear：在古英语中拼写为 eare，指的是"听觉器官"。

eye：在古英语中有两个拼写，例如麦西亚中的 ege 和撒克逊人中的 eage。

foot：源自古英语 fot。

gum：源自古英语单词 goma，指"味觉"。

hair：源自古英语 hoer。

hand：源自古英语 hond。

knee：源自古英语 cneo, cneow。

lip：源自古英语 lippa。

liver：其在古英语中拼写为 life，意思是"身体的分泌器官"。

lung：在古英语中，它是 lungen，因相比于心、胃等其他内脏器官而言，肺较轻，且能在水中浮起来，因此意为"轻器官"。

neck：在古英语中，它是 hnecca，表示"脖子，尤指颈背"。

表示概念的词

发烧：它是由晚期英语中的 fefor 演变而来，它是从拉丁语 febris 借鉴而来。

（二）源自希腊语的词

在公元前 1 世纪及之后，罗马人借用了许多希腊词。随着文艺复兴的到来，英语发生了巨大的变化。古典学术的复兴，古典拉丁语和希腊语词被引入英语。早期现代英语从希腊语中获得了语法、逻辑算术、几何学、天文学和音乐类的表达。而医学术语是受希腊语影响最深的领域之一，下面的词都从希腊语借用而来。

acme：1570年从希腊文akme借来，意思是"（最高）点"。

anorexia：1598年由希腊语借入英语。由an-（没有）和orexis（食欲，欲望）组成，意思是"食欲不振"。

koma：1398年由希腊语Kolon（大肠，食肉）借入英语。

coma：1646年由希腊语koma（深度睡眠）借来。

diagnosis：1681年起在英语中用作医学术语，意思是"区分，区别"，由dia-（分开）和gignoskein（学习）组成的diagignoskein演变而来。

dyspeptic：1694年由希腊语Dypeptos借来，意思是"难以消化"，由dys-（坏）和pepto（消化）制成。

glaucoma：它在1643年由希腊语glaukoma（不透明晶状体）借入英语。

metastasis：其在1577年进入英文，源自希腊语metastasi（转移，去除变化），由meta-和histanai组成的methistanai（去除，变化）演变而来。

（三）源自拉丁语的词

拉丁语对英语的影响最早可以追溯到罗马帝国时期。随着罗马帝国的不断迅速扩张，尤其在诺曼征服后，罗马人的语言影响力进一步加深。由于诺曼入侵者使用源自古拉丁语的语言，因此不可避免地要借用拉丁语。

abscess：1543年由拉丁语abscessus（an abscess）借入英语。字面意思是"离开"，源自ab-（离开）和cedere（去）。

acute：1570年由拉丁语actus（尖锐，尖锐）引入英语，医学意义为"发烧或来去匆匆的疾病"，最早记录于1667年。

aorta：1578年由中古拉丁语aorta借入英语。该术语由亚里士多德应用于解释心脏大动脉。它的字面意思是"挂断"。

autopsy：1651年由现代拉丁语autopsia（目击者）借入英语。由autos-（自我）和opsis（景象）组成。

（四）由法语借来单词

诺曼征服后，征服者长期统治该国，因此对英语产生了深远的影响。许多法语单词，包括很多医学著作中使用的单词，都源于英语，借用于法语一直持续到现在。

由于法语本身是拉丁语的一种演变形式，因此这些借用词中的许多形式都来自希腊语，而许多拉丁语词则是从希腊语借用而来。典型的例子如 migraine（偏头痛，一种严重的头痛，通常是单侧的）。法语词 migraine 源自拉丁语 hemicrania，它是从希腊语 hemikrania（头部一侧疼痛）借用而来，由前缀 hemi-（半）和 kranion（头骨）组合而成。

hospital：1242年由古法语 hospital（招待所）借来，原意为 "shelter for the needy"（为有需要的人提供庇护）。其"病患机构"之意最早记载于1549年。

faint(adj.)：古法语 faint（软，弱，呆滞），源自 faindre 的过去分词（假装逃避责任），于1300年进入英语。该词表示"微弱之意"始于1320年。

jaundice：该词大约于1303年由古法语 Jaunisse（黄色）借用而来，jaune 表示黄色。

doctor：该词大约于1303年由古法语 doctour 借用而来，起源于中古拉丁语 doctor（宗教教师、顾问、学者）。Doct- 的词干为 docere，意思是"展示、教导"。对"医学专业人士"的提及可以追溯到1377年，直到16世纪后期才普遍使用。

benign：该词大约于1320年由古法语 benigne（好，善良），借用而来衍生自 bene（好）和 gignere（承受，产生）。

disease：该词大约于1330年由古法语 desaise 演变而来，由 des-（没有，离开）和 aise（轻松）组成。表示"疾病"之意最早记载于1393年。

anatomy：该词于1398年进入英语，源自古法语 anatomie，由 ana-（up）+ temnein（to cut）组成。"anatomy""mummy"甚至"skeleton"是莎士比亚时代的词汇。"有组织的身体结构的科学"的意思主要来自17世纪。

ambulance：该词于1809年进入英语，基于法语 hopital ambulant（字面意思是步行到医院）而来。但它的使用并不普遍，直到它的含义从"医院"转变为"在战争期间运送伤员的车辆"才被广泛使用。

（五）从德语借来的词

与拉丁语、希腊语和法语对英语医学术语的影响相比，德语在这方面的贡献源于近代。从19世纪开始，德国在科学技术上取得了长足的进步。

这种进步需要新的词汇来表示新的发现、发明、概念和物质。因此，这些医学术语由德语创造，随后才被引入英语。

aspirin：该词是德国公司创造的商标名，源自希腊语前缀 a-（不含）和拉丁语 spiraea（榆钱），这种植物的花朵或叶子中的药物加工过的酸是天然存在的。

biology：这个词是由德国博物学家 G. Reinhold Treviranus 于 1802 年从希腊语 bios（life）和 -logia（study of）中提出的，并于当年由 Lamarck 由法语作为科学术语引入。1819 年借用于英文。

chromosome：该词于 1889 年由德语 chromosom 进入英语，并由德国解剖学家 Wilhelm von Waldeyer-hartz 在 1888 年借用希腊语 chroma（颜色）和 soma（身体）创造而来。该词的由来是因为该词结构含有一种容易被碱性染料染色的物质。

gene：1911 年由德语 gen 进入英语，并由 1905 年由丹麦科学家威廉·路德维格·约翰森（Wilhelm Ludvig Johannsen，1857—1927）创造。

（六）从其他语言借来的词

从意大利语借来的词

influenza：1743 年欧洲因暴发流行性疾病，因缺乏相应表达，得以借用意大利语 influenza（流行性感冒，流行病），该词最初为"访问，影响（星星）"之意。据记载，至少从 1504 年起，该词就在意大利语中用于表示疾病的概念。

malaria：该词于 1740 年借自意大利语 mala aria，字面意思为"坏空气"，来自 mala（坏）和 aria（空气）。这种由蚊子传播的疾病曾被认为是由沼泽地区的污浊空气引起的。

从西班牙语借来的词

mosquito：该词大约在 1583 年由西班牙语 mosquito 中借来的 mosca（飞）的缩写，源自拉丁文 musca（飞）。

直接创造新词

医学科学的发展需要越来越多的词语描述新发现并解释创新过程，同时定义概念。英语具备丰富的创造词汇能力，也体现了人类思维的创造力和才能。

acupuncture：1684年由拉丁文acus（needle）和英文puncture创造而来，最初用作名词，意思是"用针刺"。该动词于1972年首次被记录。

antacid：该词是在1732年由anti-（抗）和acid（酸剂）创造而来。

三、医学术语的特征

（一）医学术语发音

语言学习者普遍觉得医学英语术语较难发音。这种现象可以解释为大部分的术语都是外来借用词汇。因此大部分词汇在融入英语的过程中需要有一个逐渐适应的过程。

1. 字母发音

c在字母a, o, u前发音为[k]，比如单词cardiac, carcinoma, leucocyte；c在字母e, i, y前发音为[s]，比如单词paracentesis, placenta, emergency。

g在字母a,o,u前发音为[g]，比如单词gastral, anticoagulation, g在字母e, i, y前发音为[dʒ]，比如单词emergency, analgesia。

字母x作为首字母时发音为[z]，比如单词xacorin, xalogen, xanthocyanopsia，当x在其他位置时，发音为[ks]，比如单词anthrax, axilla。

2. 辅音组合的发音

ch, ph和rh为辅音组合。他们通常都会为一个整体出现在单词中。比如，ch在单词choke和chest中发音为[tʃ]，但是在大多数情况下他的发音为[k]，比如单词chromosome, chronic, cholecystitis。Ph通常发音为[f]，比如单词phobia和pharmacy。Rh通常发音为[r]，比如单词rhinal和rhinalgia。

3. 双元音的发音

每个单词的开头为双辅音组合，比如cn, gn, mn, pn, ps和pt时，首字母是不发音的。然而，当他们出现在单词中间位置时，他们的发音就会有变化。

辅音组合为cn位于单词首位时，发音为[n]，比如单词cnidoblast，但在单词gastrocnemius中，它的发音就变为[kn]。

辅音组合为 gn 位于单词首位时，发音为 [n]，比如单词 gnathal，但在单词 prognosis 中，它的发音就变为 [gn]。

辅音组合为 mn 位于单词首位时，发音为 [n]，比如单词 mneme，但在单词 amnesia 中，它的发音就变为 [mn]。

辅音组合为 pn 位于单词首位时，发音为 [n]，比如单词 pneophorus 和 pneumonia，但在单词 apnea 中，它的发音就变为 [pn]。

辅音组合为 ps 位于单词首位时，发音为 [s]，比如单词 pssychalgia 和 pseudo，但在单词 apselaphesia 中，它的发音就变为 [ps]。

辅音组合为 pt 位于单词首位时，发音为 [t]，比如单词 ptyalin、ptomatopsy 和 pteridine，但在单词 hemoptysis 中，它的发音就变为 [pt]。

（二）医学术语的复数形式

医学词汇可以根据其数字形式分为几类。比如一些词汇总是单数，尤其是表示疾病的名词，即使其中一些以 -s 结尾，例如 arrhythmia, hemophilia, bronchitis, diabetes, measles, mumps, rickets 和 shingles。

有些是变数，它们的复数形式是加 -(e)s，例如 nerve、lung、muscle 等。有些借来的词有不规则的复数形式。许多从希腊语或拉丁语演变而来的名词都属于这一类。它们大多采用原始的复数形式，尽管某些单词的复数形式是通过在单数形式上添加 -(e)s 形成的。这些词在复数使用时要特别注意。

1. 以拉丁文结尾的复数示例

表 1-1-1　以拉丁语结尾的医学术语单词表

后缀		示例	
单数形式后缀	复数形式后缀	单数形式单词	复数形式单词
-a	-ae	ampulla	ampullae
		conjunctiva	conjunctiva
		maxilla	maxillae
		pleura	pleurae
		scapula	scapulae
		vertebra	vertebrae

续表

后缀		示例	
单数形式后缀	复数形式后缀	单数形式单词	复数形式单词
-um	-a	flagellum	flagella
		labium	labia
		medium	media
-us	-i	bacillus	bacilli
		bronchus	bronchi
		coccus	cocci
		focus	foci
		fungus	fungi
		nodulus	noduli
-us	-era	genus	genera
-us	-ora	corpus	corpora
		stercus	stercora
-ex	-ices/-es	apex	apices/apexes
		pollex	pollices
-ix	-ices/-es	appendix	appendices/appendixes
		cervix	cervices/cervixes
		cortex	cortices/cortexes
		varix	varices
-s	-sa	vas	vasa

2. 以希腊语结尾的复数词

表 1-1-2 以希腊语结尾的医学术语单词表

后缀		示例	
单数形式后缀	复数形式后缀	单数形式单词	复数形式单词
-ma	-mata/-s	enema	enemata/enemas
		fibroma	fibromata/fibromas
		lymphoma	lymphomata/lymphomas
		stoma	stomata/stomas

续表

后缀		示例	
单数形式后缀	复数形式后缀	单数形式单词	复数形式单词
-on	-a	encephalon	encephala
		ganglion	ganglia
		phenomenon	phenomena
-is	-es	analysis	analyses
		arthrosis	arthroses
		crisis	crises
		dermatosis	dermatoses
		epiphysis	epiphyses
		neurosis	neuroses
		paralysis	paralyses
-is	-ides	epididymis	epididymides
		glottis	glottides
-ax	-aces/-es	thorax	thoraces/thoraxes
-inx	-iges	meninx	meninges

（三）医学术语的同义现象

正如前面所讨论的，医学术语来自不同的起源，包括古英语、拉丁语、希腊语、法语和其他语言。这种起源多样性的一个结果是不同的元素甚至词被用来指代相同的概念、事物或想法。例如，body 一词源自古英语 bodig，原意为"木桶"。后来英语借用拉丁语 corpus 等词来表示"身体"，包括 corporal, corpuscle, corpse。从希腊语中，英语借用 soma 表示"身体"，它被用作许多相关词的形成元素，如 somatic, somatocyte, somatology 和 somatoscopy。

另一个很好的例子是表示"心脏"的词。heart 来自古英语 heorte。从拉丁语中，英语借用了 cor（heart），其意是核心和亲切；并从希腊语 cardia（希腊语中的 kardia）带来了 cardiology, cardiac, cardiovascular。以下虽然不是详尽无遗，但列出了不同来源的同义词构建元素。

表1-1-3 医学术语起源示例表

所指部位	原始语言或其他语言	拉丁语起源	希腊语起源
body	bodig	corpus: corporal	soma: somatic
bowel	bouele（french）	intestine: intestinal	entero: enteron
breath	broe	respire: respiratory	pneuma: pneumatometer
fat	foett	adip-: adipofibroma	lipo-: lipocyte
hand	hond	manus: manual	cheiro-, chiro-: cheiroplasty, chiroplasty
heart	heorte	cor-:core	cardia-: cardiocentesis
joint	joint	artic-: articulation	arthr-: arthrocele
kidney	kidenere	ren-: renal	nephron-: nephritis
navel	nafela	umbilicus: umbilicular	omphalos: ompjalecele
red	read	rub-: rubeosis	erythro-: erythrocatalysis
skin	skinn	cutis: subcutaneous	derma: epidermis
tongue	tungue	lingua-: lingual	glossa: glossal
vessel	vessel	vas: vascular	angio-: angiology
woman	wimman	fem-: female	gyn-: gynaecology

四、医学术语构词法

医学术语主要由四大构词要素构成，即词根、前缀、后缀和现存词。一般来说，医学术语有七个常用的构词法。它们是词缀法、复合法、转化法、拼缀法、逆生法、截短法和首字母简略词法等。

（一）词缀法

词缀是指通过前缀和后缀组合构成词的一种方法。它包括前缀和后缀。词缀法是将一个词缀加在词根前面的形态学过程。通常词缀倾向于语义导向，即在词性不变的情况下给词根增加新的意义。例如，autograft, isograft, allograft, xenograft都具有相同的词根graft, 但由于前缀不同而表示不同类型的移植物。Intracranial, antiallergenic, restenosis, asymptomatic, antineoplastic, nondiabetic, hyperlipidemi, heterogeneous都属于这类词。

第一章 医学英语术语学

后缀是一种形态学过程，其中后缀附加到词根的末端。与前缀不同，后缀倾向于改变单词的词性。例如，immunity，immunity，immunize 和 immunization 都有基本的含义，都与生物体的"免疫"有关，但属于不同的词类。Immune，immunity，immunize 和 immunization 等其他词都是改变后缀构成的。

当两个词根组合或后缀连接到一个词根时，如果没有元音连接这两种形式，则需要添加一个元音，并将这种组合形式称为组合元音。最常用的组合元音是 o，或者是 -oi-，-oa-。下面列举前缀构词法：

前缀 + 词根

inject：in-（前缀，into）+jec（t）（词根，to throw）

前缀 + 连接元音 + 词根

ectoderm：ect（前缀，outside）+ derm-（词根，a condition of）

词根 + 后缀

stasis：sta（词根，to stand）+-sis（后缀，a condition of）

词根 + 连接元音 + 后缀

sclerosis：scler-（词根，to harden）+sis（后缀，a condition of）

前缀 + 词根 + 后缀

perirenal：peri-（前缀，around）+ren（词根，kidney）+-al（后缀，pertaining to）

前缀 + 词根 + 连接元音 + 后缀

synarthrosis：syn-（前缀，together）+arthr-（词根，joint）+o（连接元音）+-sis（后缀，acondition of）

前缀 + 前缀 + 词根 + 连接元音 + 后缀

contraindication：contra-（前缀，against）+in-（前缀，toward）+dic(t)（词根，to speak）+-tion（后缀，the action or process involved）

词根 + 词根 + 后缀

sialadenitis：sial-（词根，saliva）+aden-（词根，gland）+-it is（后缀，an inflammatory condition）

词根 + 连接元音 + 词根 + 后缀

hemophilia：hem（词根，-blood）+o（连接元音）+phil-（词根，

第一部分 医学英语

beloved)+-ia(后缀, pathological 偶然 abnormal condition)。

前缀+词根+词根+后缀

hyperglycemia: hyper-(前缀, excessive)+glyc(词根, sweet)+(h)em-(后缀, blood)+-ia(后缀, condition)。

(二)复合法

复合法通常是连接两个或多个单词来形成新的单词的过程。以这种方式构成的词称为复合词。基于拼写特征的复合词可分为三种类型。第一种是开放式复合词。之所以这样叫，是因为一个开放式复合词由两个或多个单独书写的单词组成，例如 woman doctor, man nurse, sleeping sickness, brain death, family planning, birth control, gray matter 和 white matter。带连字符的复合词由两个或多个由连字符连接的词组成，例如 high-resolution, host-specific, deaf-mute, air-borne, bottle-feed 和 graft-versus-host。固定复合词由两个单词组合成一个词的，例如 windpipe, sleepwalk, overweight 和 nosebleed。

在医学语言中，复合法还有一种特殊的构词形式，即新古典复合构词法，其在形成新的医学词方面发挥着越来越重要的作用，因此值得关注。新古典复合构词法是指从古典语言（拉丁语和希腊语）的元素中创造出来的复合词。这些词既不是古典拉丁语，也不是希腊语。相反，它们是通过将源自经典语言的元素组合在一起而形成的。比如，biocide, lysosome, bio-science, psychanalysis, biophysics 和 chemotherapy 等词都是新古典复合构词法产生的词汇。

(三)转化法

转化在形成新词方面非常有效。转化法即为一个词形成过程，在这个过程中，一个词在不改变形式的情况下被转换成一个新的类别。例如，e-mail 最初被用作名词，即"电子邮件"。在医学术语中，一个很好的例子就是 stent。其他的词汇包括 love, taste, smell, skin, plaster, mask, faint 和 empty，都可以将其名词转化为动词。

(四)拼缀法

拼缀法指将两个单词的部分拼缀到一起组合成新的单词。在这个过程中，一般有三种形式。

· 14

part+part　　　　　genome（gene+chromosome）

whole+part　　　　breathalyzer（breath+analyzer）

part+whole　　　　Medicare（medical+care）

（五）逆生法

逆生法指的是通过添加后缀，将现有动词转换成名词形式。比如 teacher 由 teach 和后缀 -er 组成。也就是说，动词是通过删除表面或想象词缀由现有名词构成而来。例如，chain-smoke 来自 chainssmoker，而 automate 来自 automation。其他通过逆生构词法产生的医学术语包括 diagnose 来源于 diagnosis，ovulate 来源于 ovulation，palpitate 来源于 palpitation，injure 来源于 injury 等。

（六）截短法

截短法也称为缩短法，指的是一个单词被去掉部分形式而不改变其原有的意义和属性。比如说，exam 即由 examination 而来，flu 来自 influenza，specs 来自 spectacles，psych 来自 psychology。

（七）首字母简略词法

首字母简略词在医学文献中很常见。首字母简略词是由一组词的首字母组合而来的单词。该构词法一直被广泛使用，单词数量一直在增加，尤其是在科学和技术方面。医学文献中创造了大量的缩略词，如 CT（computer tomography），RBC（red blood cell），C.C（chief complaint），BMR（basal metabolic rate），B.P（blood pressure），GP（general practitioner），NP（nurse practitioner）等。

某些首字母简略词不是由复合词的单个词的首字母组成。相反，它们主要由单词的首字母加上同一单词的其他组成部分的首字母组成，例如 TB（tuberculosis），OD（overdose），IV（intravenous），NP（neuropsychiatry）。

在学习过程中，我们还应该注意不是来自现代英语而是来自拉丁语或希腊语的缩略词。以下是此类中最常用的首字母缩略词。

a.c.（ante cibum = before meal）

p.c.（post cibum=after meal）

b.i.d（bis in die= twice a day）

t.i.d(ter in die=three times a day)

i.d(quarter in die=four times a day)

b.i.n(bis in nocte=twice a night)

O.D.(oculus dexter=right eye)

O.S.(oculus sinister=left eye)

p.r.n.(pro re nata=as needed)

q.h(quaque hora=every hour)

q.m(quaque mane=every morning)

q.n(quaque nocte=every night)

(八)类推法

类推法在构词中也起着越来越重要的作用。类推即是通过新创造的词和现有的对应词之间的类比来创造一个新词的过程。在医学术语中，myalgia就是一个很好的例子。它是为了类比已经存在的neuralgia(神经痛)而创造的。以这种方式创建的其他医学术语包括以genomics(基因组学)为模型的proteomics，metabomics和transcriptomics，以neurotic为模型的psychotic，以progress为模型的retrogress，以及以epidemic为模型的pandemic。

五、词根和组合形式

词根是单词中所有添加的元素都被删除后不可再分的部分。词根是一个词的核心和最基本含义。医学术语的其他语义元素由前缀和后缀提供。

词根可以独立存在并具有意义。它还能够与其他组成部分结合形成一个有意义的医学术语。例如，derm是一个词根，表示"皮肤"。它可以单独作为一个词来指代"皮肤"。它还可以与其他组合产生其他词。如epidermis, dermis, dermatology, dermatitis, dermatosis, dermatoid等。

如果词根与后缀或另一个词根组合，则通常使用组合元音。具有组合元音的词根称为组合形式。此外"o"和"a"也用作组合元音。

aden/o：腺体　　　　　　*aden*ocarcinoma 腺癌

angi/o：血管　　　　　　*angi*oplasty 血管成形术

arthr/o：关节　　　　　　*arthro*centesis 关节穿刺术

cardio/o：心脏　　　　　*cardio*megaly 心脏肥大
cerebr/o：脑　　　　　　*cerebro*vascular 脑血管
chondr/o：软骨　　　　　*chondro*dystrophis 软骨营养不良
crain/o：颅骨　　　　　 *cranio*schisis 颅骨骨折
dermat/o：皮肤　　　　　*dermat*itis 皮炎
epitheli/o：上皮　　　　*epithelio*ma 上皮瘤
fibr/o：纤维　　　　　　*fibro*myositis 纤维肌炎
gastr/o：胃　　　　　　 *gastro*ptosis 胃下垂
hepat/o：肝　　　　　　 *hepato*megaly 肝肥大
lymph/o：淋巴　　　　　 *lympho*cyte 淋巴细胞
mamm/o-：胸部　　　　　 *mammo*plasia 乳腺增生
nephr/o：肾脏　　　　　 *nephro*megaly 肾肿大
neur/o：神经　　　　　　*neur*itis 神经炎
ocul/o：眼睛　　　　　　*oculo*pathy 眼病
ophthalm/o：眼睛　　　　*ophthalmo*neuritis 眼神经炎
oste/o：骨头　　　　　　*osteo*malacia 骨软化症
pleur/o：胸膜　　　　　 *pleuro*dynia 胸膜痛
ren/o：肾脏　　　　　　 *reno*pathy 肾病
rhin/o：鼻子　　　　　　*rhino*rrhagia 鼻出血
stern/o：胸骨　　　　　 *sterno*schisis 胸骨劈裂
thorac/o：胸部　　　　　*thoraco*schisis 胸裂
ur/o：尿　　　　　　　　*ur*emia 尿毒症

六、前缀

前缀是放在单词或组合词之前的字母或字母组合，以改变或修饰单词的基本意义，这种造词过程称为前缀法。大部分前缀描述了空间关系。一部分表示否定概念，还有一些描述物体或概念的物理特性或属性。在表示空间关系的前缀中，有的成对表示相反的关系，例如ab-(远离)和ad-(向)，而其他的则不成对。

第一部分 医学英语

（一）配对空间前缀

表1-1-4 拉丁语配对空间前缀表

前缀	举例
ad-（toward） ab-（away from）	*ad*duct *ab*duct
af-（toward） ef-（away from）	*af*ferent *ef*ferent
ante-（forward, before） retro-（backward）	*ante*brachium *retro*cervical
anter/o-（farther forward） poster/o-（farther back）	*anter*ior *poster*ior
dextr/o-（on the right side） sinistro-（on the left side）	*dextro*cardia *sinistro*cular
extra/o-（outside of, beyond） intra/o-（inside, within）	*extra*celluar *intra*celluar
infer-（lower） super-（above, over, higher）	*infer*ior *super*ior
infra-（inferior to, below, or beneath） supra-（above，over）	*infra*costal *supra*costal
pron-（bend forward） supine-（lying on the back）	*pron*e *supine*
pro-（before, forward） ap/o-（from, away from）	*pro*state *apo*crine

表1-1-5 希腊语配对空间前缀表

前缀	举例
ana-（up, back） *cata*-（down, down from）	*ana*bolism *cata*bolism
hyper-（over, above, beyond; excessive） *hypo*-（beneath, under）	*hyper*calcium *hypo*dermis
endo-（inside, inner） *exo*-（out of, outside）	*endo*scope *exo*thermic

(二) 非配对空间前缀

表1-1-6　拉丁语非配对空间前缀表

前缀	举例
circum-（around, encircling）	*circum*flex
co-（with, together）	*co*enzyme
contra-（against, the opposite side or direction）	*contra*lateral
de-（down from, away from, off）	*de*congestant
dif-（apart, separate）	*dif*fuse
dis-（apart, separate）	*dis*location
en-（in, on, within）	*en*cysted
epi-（upon, above, or beside）	*epi*dermis
in-（in, into, on, toward, against）	*in*flate
ob-（against, in the way of）	*ob*struction
per-（through, throughout）	*per*forate
re-（back, again）	*re*generation
sub-（under）	*sub*arachnoid
syn-（with, together, fused）	*syn*arthrosis
trans-（across, through, beyond, over）	*trans*cutaneous
ultra-（beyond）	*ultra*violet

表1-1-7　希腊语非配对空间前缀表

前缀	举例
anti-（against, opposing）	*anti*arrhythmic
dia-（through, thorough, apart）	*dia*gnosis, diarrhea
ecto-（outside of, outer）	*ecto*derm
mes/o-（in the middle of, intermediate, moderate）	*mes*encephalon
meta-（change, beyond, after）	*meta*stasis
pali-（backward, again）	*pali*ngraphia
para-（beside, by the side of, beyond）	*para*lgesia
peri-（around）	*peri*natal
tele-（far away, at a distance）	*tele*pathy

第一部分　医学英语

(三) 否定前缀

否定前缀，顾名思义，赋予词汇否定意义。

表 1-1-8　表示否定的前缀表

前缀	举例
a-/an-（not, without, absence of）	*a*sepsis, *an*emia
de-（do or make the opposite of; reverse）	*de*fibrillation, *de*hydration
dis-/dys-（not, the converse of）	*dis*able, *dys*pepsia
in-/im-（not）	*im*balance
non-（not）	*non*infectious
un-（not）	*non*viable, *un*saturated

(四) 数字前缀

在前缀中不可忽视的有一部分表示数量的前缀。其中还有一部分不同表现形式但却表示同样含义的数量前缀，存在这一现象的主要原因在于这些前缀的起源不同。

表 1-1-9　表示数字的前缀表

前缀	举例
nulli-（zero, nothing）	*nulli*para
semi-（half, partly, partially）	*semi*permeable
hemi-（half, partly, partially）	*hemi*plegia
uni-（one, a single, alone）	*uni*lateral
mono-（one, single, alone）	*mono*cyte
haplo-（simple, simply; single; once）	*haplo*id
bi-（two, twice）	*bi*ceps
ambi-（both）	*ambi*dexterity
amphi-（both, on both sides）	*amphi*centric
di-（two, twice, double, divide）	*di*cephalus
diplo-（double）	*diplo*pia
ter-（thrice, threefold）	*ter*oxide
tri-（three, third, thrice, triple）	*tri*glyceride
quadri-, quadru-, quadr-	*quadri*ceps

续表

前缀	举例
tetra-（four）	*tetra*plegia
quint-（five, fifth）	*quint*uplet
deca-（ten）	*deca*gram
deci-（tenth）	*deci*meter
centi-（one hundred）	*centi*grade
hect-, hector-（one hundred）	*hect*ogram
kilo-（thousand）	*kilo*calorie
nano-, nanno-（one billionth of a gram）	*nano*gram
pauc-（few）	*pauc*ity
oligo-（little, few）	*olig*uria
poly-（much, many）	*poly*uria
plur-（more than one）	*plur*icellular
multi-（much, many）	*multi*para
holo-（whole）	*holo*enzyme
pan-（all）	*pan*cytopenia

（五）颜色前缀

表 1-1-10 表示颜色的前缀表

前缀	举例
alb/i-, albino/o-, album/o-（white）	*alb*ino
chloro-（green）	*chloro*pia
cirrho-（tawny）	*cirrho*sis
cyan/o-（dark blue）	*cyan*osis
erythr/o-（red）	*erythr*ocyte
glauc/o-（gray）	*glauc*oma
leuk/o-, leuc/o-（white）	*leuk*ocyte
melan/o-（black, dark）	*melan*ocyte
polio-（gray）	*polio*sis
purpur-（purple）	*purpur*a
rub-, rubi-, rube/o-（red）	*rub*escent
xanth/o-（yellow）	*xantho*derma

（六）其他前缀

表 1-1-11　其他形式的前缀表

前缀	举例
acro-（extremity of the body; height; top）	*acro*cyanosis
auto-（self, independently）	*auto*matic
brachy-（short）	*brachy*dactyly
brady-（slow）	*brady*pnea
dys-（difficult, impaired, abnormal）	*dys*graphia
eu-（good, well, easy）	*eu*genics
hetero-（other, different）	*hetero*generous
homo-, homeo-, homio-（same, like）	*homo*graft
hydro-（water）	*hydro*pericardium
iso-（equal, alike, the same, or uniform）	*iso*enzyme
macro-（large, long, extensive）	*macro*glossia
mal-（bad, abnormal）	*mal*absorption
micro-（small）	*micro*be
tachy-（swift, rapid）	*tachy*rhythmia

七、后缀

后缀是指附加到词根后面以更改词根的含义或词的类别。医学语言中的后缀分为简单后缀和复合后缀两种。简单后缀是那些没有添加任何其他内容的后缀。例如，-itis 是简单后缀，意思是"炎症"，比如 nephritis（肾炎）和 hepatitis（肝炎）。复合后缀通常是基本后缀和简单后缀的组合。例如，-pathy 是一个复合后缀，由基本的 patho-（疾病、痛苦）和简单的后缀 -y（条件、行为、过程）连接而成。因此复合后缀 -pathy 表示"疾病或患病状况"，比如 nephropathy 肾病。

复合后缀也可包含前缀。比如 -ectomy，它是前缀 ec-（出去），词根是 tom-（切除）和简单后缀 -y（行动，过程）的组合。因此，-ectomy 指的是手术切除、或切除的过程，如 tonsillectomy（扁桃体切除术）、appendectomy（阑尾切除术）和 thyroidectomy（甲状腺切除术）。

（一）简单后缀

医学术语简单后缀可大致分为两部分，即名词形式后缀和形容词后缀。

1. 名词形式简单后缀

表 1-1-12　名词形式简单后缀表

后缀	举例
-*ary*（indicating a person or place）	capill*ary*
-*e*（an instrument）	microtom*e*
-*escence*（state）	adol*escence*
-*ia*（condition, quality, entity）	hydrophob*ia*
-*ice*（study of, name of a science）	obstr*ics*
-(*s/t*) *ion*（describing the act or action; condition; process）	palpita*tion*
-*ism*（action, or its results; a system of theory or practice）	embol*ism*
-*ist*（agent of an action; practitioner of a profession or art）	pediatr*ist*
-*itis*（inflammatory condition）	hepat*itis*, tonsill*itis*
-*ity*（state, quality）	abnormal*ity*
-(*i*) *um*（referring to part in relation to a whole）	pericard*ium*
-*ment*（the result or product of an action, or the means or instrument of an action）	nourish*ment*
-*oma*（tumor or morbid growth）	lymph*oma*
-*osis*（a condition, usually abnormal or pathological）	thromb*osis*
-*sy*（the action or the result of this）	biop*sy*
-*ure*（action or process or the result of this）	sut*ure*

2. 形容词形式简单后缀

表 1-1-13　形容形式简单后缀表

后缀	举例
-*ac*（pertaining to）	ili*ac*
-*aceous*（having the qualities or nature of）	seb*aceous*
-*al*（pertaining to, relating to）	dent*al*, ren*al*
-*ar*（pertaining to, belonging to）	cellul*ar*
-*ary*（pertaining to, belonging to）	cili*ary*
-*eal*（pertaining to, relating to）	esophag*eal*
-*form*（resembling）	denti*form*
-*ic*（pertaining to）	opt*ic*

第一部分　医学英语

续表

后缀	举例
-il（e）（characterized by）	sterile
-ine（of the nature of, pertaining to）	bovine
-ive（characterized by）	adoptive
-ode（resembling）	nematode
-oid（resembling,）	cystoid
-ory（characterized by, pertaining to）	sensory
-ous（pertaining to, or containing, or secreting）	mucous

（二）复合后缀

复合后缀由一个词根和一个简单的后缀组成，医学术语构词中起着至关重要的作用。复合后缀可分为三种类型，即解剖生理相关后缀、病理相关后缀和手术或治疗相关后缀

1. 解剖学和生理学后缀

解剖学和生理学后缀是指解剖学、生理学或组织学结构或正常的身体功能的后缀。

表1-1-14　表示解剖学和生理学意义的后缀表

后缀	举例
-cele（cavity, belly, hollow）	blastocele
-cyte（cell）	phagocyte, astrocyte
-esthesia（a condition of felling, perception, or sensation）	anesthesia
-genic（causing, forming, or producing）	pyogenic
-genesis（formation; the production or procreation）	odontogenesis
-poiesis（the making or production of）	hemopoiesis

2. 病理后缀

表1-1-15　表示病理意义的后缀表

后缀	举例
-algia（pain, painful condition）	arthralgia
-cele（hernia, protrusion, distension）	diaphragmatocele

续表

后缀	举例
-*ectasia*（a condition of dilation, extension）	arteri*ectasia*
-*ectasis*（a condition of dilation, extension）	atel*ectasis*
-*emia*（a pecified condition of the blood）	ur*emia*
-*iasis*（a condition, formation of）	cholelith*iasis*
-*lysis*（a breaking down, loosening）	cyto*lysis*
-*malacia*（the softening or softness of a tissue）	osteo*malacia*
-*megaly*（an enlargement of a part of the body）	spleno*megaly*
-*odynia*（a state of pain）	pleur*odynia*
-*paresis*（slight or incomplete paralysis）	hemi*paresis*
-*penia*（a deficiency, lack）	erythro*penia*
-*phasia*（a manner of speaking）	dys*phasia*
-*philia*（a tendency towards an action or activity, an abnormal liking or appetite for a thing）	hemo*philia*
-*phobia*（a condition of formation or development）	claustro*phobia*
-*plasia*（a condition of formation or development）	dys*plasia*
-*plegia*（paralysis, stroke）	quadri*plegia*
-*ptosis*（a prolapse or downward displacement of an organ or organs）	entero*ptosis*
-(r)*rhagia*（a fluid discharge or excessive quantity）	leuko*rrhagia*
-*rrhea*（a fluid discharge of）	dia*rrhea*
-*rrhexis*（a rupture of a part of the body）	hepato*rrhexis*
-*sclerosis*（morbid hardening）	arterio*sclerosis*
-*schisis*（a cleft or cleavage）	cheilo*schisis*
-*spasm*（convulsion）	entero*spasm*
-*stenosis*（an abnormal narrowing of the larynx）	laryngo*stenosis*

3. 外科手术和治疗后缀

表 1-1-16　表示外科手术和治疗的后缀表

后缀	举例
-*centesis*（surgical puncture to withdraw fluid）	para*centesis*
-*clysis*（washing）	colo*clysis*

续表

后缀	举例
-desis (binding, stabilization, fusion)	arthro*desis*
-etomy (the surgical removal, excision)	append*ectomy*
-gram (a drawing, record, piece of writing)	electroencephalo*gram*
-graph (a machine or instrument for making or for reproducing or transmitting something written or drawn)	thermo*graphy*
-iatry (branch of medicine; a type of medical treatment or healing)	psych*iatry*
-meter (an instrument used in measuring)	thermo*meter*
-metery (the process, art, or science of measuring something)	calori*metry*
-pexis (a surgical fixation or a neutralization)	spleno*pexy*
-plasty (surgical shaping or molding)	labio*plasty*
-rrhaphy (s suturing in place)	cardio*rrhaphy*
-scope (a machine or instrument for observing or viewing with the eye)	ophthalmo*scope*
-scopy (the art or process of observation in a manner)	radio*scopy*
-stomy (a surgical opening)	colo*stomy*
-tomy (a surgical incision)	litho*tomy*
-tome (an instrument for cutting; a segment, region)	derma*tome*
-tripsy (crushing)	litho*tripsy*

4. 其他后缀

表 1-1-17　表示其他意义的后缀表

后缀	举例
-blast (a bud or budding)	osteo*blast*
-clast (breaking, destroying)	osteo*clast*
-pathy (a suffering, or illness)	cardio*pathy*
-phagia, -phagy (eating, ingesting, swallowing)	dys*phagia*
-stasis, -stasia (standing still, stoppage)	meta*stasis*
-uria (the presence of a substance in urine)	achromat*uria*
-vorous (of or referring to feeding on)	herbi*vorous*

第二章　各系统术语

一、皮肤系统

（一）皮肤系统词根和组合形式

表 1-2-1　表示皮肤系统词根和组合形式表

皮肤系统词根和组合形式	举例
acanth/o-（thorny, spiny）	*acanth*oid [əˈkænθɔɪd] 刺状的；棘状的；针棘状；棘样的
hidr/o-（sweat）	*hidr*orrhea [hɪdrɒˈrɪə] 多汗
histi/o-（tissue）	*histo*lysis [hɪsˈtɒlɪsɪs] 组织溶解
ichthy/o-（fish）	*ichthy*osis [ˌɪkθɪˈəʊsɪs] 鱼鳞癣
lact/o-（milk）	*lacto*protein [ˌlæktəʊˈprəʊtiːn] 乳蛋白质
myc/o-, myet-（fungus）	*myco*sis [maɪˈkəʊsɪs] 霉菌病
onych/o-（nail）	*onycho*malacia [ɒnaɪkɒməˈleɪʃə] 甲软化
pachy/o-（thick, cogged）	*pachy*derma [pæˈkɪdɜːmə] 皮肥厚
pil/o-（hair）	*pilo*sebaceous [paɪləʊsɪˈbeɪʃəs] 毛囊皮脂的
seb-（suet）	*seb*orrhea [sɪbɒrˈhɪə] 皮脂溢
squam/o-（squama）	*squam*ous [ˈskweɪməs] 鳞状的
thel/o-（nipple）	*thel*itis [θɪˈlaɪtɪs] 乳头炎
trich/o-（hair）	*trich*oid [ˈtrɪkɒɪd] 毛发状的
xer/o-（dry, dryness）	*xero*derma [ˌzɪərəʊˈdɜːmə] 干皮病

（二）皮肤系统临床和病理术语

1. 皮肤系统炎症和感染的术语

表 1-2-2　表示皮肤系统炎症和感染的术语表

皮肤系统炎症和感染术语	中文释义
acne	[ˈækni] 痤疮
athlete's foot	[ˈæθliːt fʊt] 足癣
carbuncle	[ˈkɑːbʌŋkl] 痈
cellulitis	[ˌseljʊˈlaɪtɪs] 蜂窝组织炎
chilblain	[ˈtʃɪlbleɪn] 冻疮
dermatitis	[ˌdɜːməˈtaɪtɪs] 皮炎；皮肤炎
dermatographia	[dəˌmætəˈɡræfɪə] 皮肤画纹现象
dermatophytosis	[ˈdɜːmətəʊfaɪˈtəʊsɪs] 脚气；脚癣；皮真菌病
eczema	[ˈeksmə; ˈeksɪmə] 湿疹
erysipelas	[ˌerɪˈsɪpɪləs] 丹毒
felon	[ˈfelən] 瘭疽
frostbite	[ˈfrɒstbaɪt] 冻伤，冻疮
furunculosis	[fjʊˌrʌŋkjʊˈləʊsɪs] 疖病
herpes	[ˈhɜːpiːz] 疱疹
impetigo	[ˌɪmpɪˈtaɪɡəʊ] 脓疱病
onychomycosis	[ɒnɪkəʊmaɪˈkəʊsɪs] 甲癣，甲真菌病
parakeratosis	[ˈpærəˌkerəˈtəʊsɪs] 角化不全
paronychia	[ˌpærəˈnɪkɪə] 甲沟炎
pediculosis	[pɪˌdɪkjʊˈləʊsɪs] 生虱子，虱病
scabies	[ˈskeɪbiːz] 疥疮
tinea	[ˈtɪnɪə] 癣
urticaria	[ˌɜːtɪˈkeərɪə] 荨麻疹；风团
wart	[wɔːt] 疣
wheal	[hwiːl] 水疱

2. 皮肤系统病理术语

表 1-2-3　表示皮肤系统病理术语表

皮肤系统病理术语	中文释义
albinism	[ˈælbɪnɪzəm] 白化病；皮肤变白症
alopecia	[ˌæləˈpiːʃə] 脱发（症），秃头（症）
anhidrosis	[ˌænhɪˈdrəʊsɪs] 无汗症；汗缺乏
bedsore	[ˈbedsɔː(r)] 褥疮
bulla	[ˈbʊlə] 大疱
callosity	[kəˈlɒsɪtɪ] 老茧皮；硬结
chloasma	[kləʊˈæzmə] 黄褐斑
cicatrix	[ˈsɪkətrɪks] 瘢痕，伤痕
cyanosis	[ˌsaɪəˈnəʊsɪs] 发绀，青紫
dermatofibroma	[ˌdɜːmətəfaɪˈbrəʊmə] 皮肤纤维瘤
dermatosis	[ˌdɜːməˈtəʊsɪs] 皮肤病
dyskeratosis	[diːzkərəˈtəʊsɪs] 角化不良，角化病
ecchymosis	[ˌekɪˈməʊsɪs] 瘀斑
epithelioma	[ˌepɪˌθiːlɪˈəʊmə] 上皮瘤；上皮癌
erythema	[ˌerɪˈθiːmə] 红斑，红疹
exanthema	[ˌeksænˈθiːmə] 疹
gangrene	[ˈɡæŋɡriːn] 坏疽
hidradenoma	[ˌhaɪdrædɪˈnəʊmə] 汗腺腺瘤
hirsutism	[ˈhɜːsjuːˌtɪzəm] 多毛症
hyperhidrosis	[ˌhaɪpəhɪˈdrəʊsɪs] 多汗（症）；剧汗
hyperkeratosis	[ˌhaɪpəˌkerəˈtəʊsɪs] 角化过度；眼角膜细胞增多
ichthyosis	[ˌɪkθɪˈəʊsɪs] 鱼鳞癣
keloid	[ˈkiːlɔɪd] 瘢痕疙瘩，瘢痕瘤
macula	[ˈmækjʊlə]（视网膜）黄斑；（皮肤上的）斑点，色斑
melanoma	[ˌmeləˈnəʊmə] 黑素瘤；胎记瘤
nevus	[ˈniːvəs] 痣
nodule	[ˈnɒdjuːl] 小结；小瘤；节结
pallor	[ˈpælə(r)] 苍白
papule	[ˈpæpjuːl] 丘疹
pemphigus	[ˈpemfɪɡəs] 天疱疮
pruritus	[prʊˈraɪtəs] 瘙痒，瘙痒症

续表

皮肤系统病理术语	中文释义
psoriasis	[səˈraɪəsɪs] 牛皮癣；银屑癣
purpura	[ˈpɜːpjʊrə] 紫癜
pustule	[ˈpʌstjuːl] 脓疱
scale	[skeɪl] 皮屑
scar	[skɑː(r)] 伤疤
squamous	[ˈskweɪməs] 鳞状的；有鳞的；鳞部的
ulcer	[ˈʌlsə(r)] 溃疡
vesicle	[ˈvesɪkl] 泡，囊；水疱
vitiligo	[ˌvɪtɪˈlaɪɡəʊ] 白癜风
xanthoma	[zænˈθəʊmə] 黄瘤；黄色瘤；黄疣
xeroderma	[ˌzɪərə(ʊ)ˈdɜːmə] 干皮病；皮肤干燥病

（三）皮肤系统检查术语

表1-2-4　表示皮肤系统检查术语表

皮肤系统检查术语	中文释义
autodermic graft	自皮移植物；自体真皮移植片
buccal smear	口腔黏膜涂片
dermabrasion	[ˌdɜːməˈbreɪʒən] 磨去皮肤疤痕手术
heterodermic graft	异体皮移植术
patch test	皮肤过敏试验
scratch test	过敏性测验
skin graft	植皮手术

（四）皮肤系统药学术语

表1-2-5　表示皮肤系统药学术语表

皮肤系统药学术语	中文释义
antibacterial	[ˌæntɪbækˈtɪərɪəl] 抗菌药
antifungal	[ˌæntɪˈfʌŋɡəl] 抗真菌药
anti-infective	[ˌæntɪɪnˈfektɪv] 抗感染药
antipruritic	[ˌæntɪprʊəˈrɪtɪk] 止痒剂

续表

皮肤系统药学术语	中文释义
antiseptic	[ˌæntɪˈseptɪk] 防腐剂，抗菌剂
astringent	[əˈstrɪndʒənt] 收敛剂；止血药
keratolytic	[ˌkerətəˈlɪtɪk] 角质层分离的，促成脱皮的
parasiticide	[ˌpærəˈsɪtɪˌsaɪd] 驱虫剂
topical corticosteroid	[ˌkɔːtɪkəʊˈstɪərɒɪd] 局部皮质类固醇

二、骨骼系统

（一）骨骼系统词根、后缀和组合形式

表 1-2-6　表示骨骼系统词根、后缀和组合形式表

骨骼系统词根、组合形式（后缀）	中文释义
ankyl/o-（crooked, bent, stiff）	*ankylo*ses [ˈæŋkɪləʊsɪz] 关节强硬
carp/o-（wrist）	*carpo*metacarpal [kɑːɒmetəˈkɑːpl] 腕掌的
caud/o-（tail, lower part of the body）	*caud*al [ˈkɔːdl] 尾部的
cleid/o-（calvicle）	*cleido*cranial [klɪaɪˈdɒkrənɪəl] 锁骨头颅的
dactyl/o-（finger）	*dactylo*lysis [ˌdæktɪˈlɒlɪsɪs] 指脱落
ili/o-（ilium or flank）	*ilio*lumbar [ɪlaɪəˈlʌmbər] 髂腰的
ischi/o-（hip）	*ischio*dynia [ɪstˈʃaɪdɪnɪə] 坐骨神经痛的
lamin/o-（lamina）	*lamin*ectomy [ˌlæmɪˈnektəmɪ] 椎板切除术
lumb/o-（loins）	*lumbo*dorsal [lʌˈbəʊdɔːsl] 腰背的
maxilla/o-（maxilla）	*maxill*itis [mækˈsɪlaɪtɪs] 上颌骨炎
osse/o-（bone）	*osseo*fibrous [ˈɒsefɪbrəs] 骨纤维组织的
rachi/o-（spine）	*rachi*centesis [ˈrəʃɪsəntɪzɪs] 椎管穿刺法
scapho-（boat-shaped）	*scapho*id [ˈskæfɔɪd] 舟状骨
scapul/o-（scapula, shoulder blade）	*scapulo*pexy [skæpjʊləˈpeksɪ] 肩胛固定术
scoli/o-（twisted orcrooked）	*scolio*sis [skəʊlɪˈəʊsɪs] 脊柱侧凸
spondyl/o-（vertebra）	*spondylo*dynia [ˌspɒndɪləʊˈdɪnjə] 脊椎病
syndesm/o-（ligament）	*syndesmo*tomy [sɪndzməʊˈtəmɪ] 韧带切开术
vertebr/o-（vertebra）	*vertebr*ectomy [vɜːtɪbˈrektəmɪ] 椎骨切除术
-physis（to grow）	epi*physis* [ɪˈpɪfɪsɪs] 骺；脑上体；松果体
-porosis（passage, pore）	osteo*porosis* [ˌɒstɪəʊpəˈrəʊsɪs] 骨质疏松症

（二）骨骼系统临床和病理术语

1. 骨骼系统炎症和感染的术语

表 1-2-7　表示骨骼系统炎症和感染的术语表

骨骼系统炎症和感染的术语	中文释义
arthritis	[ɑːˈθraɪtɪs] 关节炎
bursitis	[ˌbɜːˈsaɪtɪs] 黏液囊炎
caries	[ˈkeəriːz] 龋齿；骨疡；骨溃疡
coxitis	[kɔkˈsaɪtɪs] 髋关节炎
epiphysitis	[epɪfɪˈsaɪtɪs] 骨骺炎
osteitis	[ˌɒstɪˈaɪtɪs] 骨炎
osteoarthritis	[ˌɒstɪəʊɑːˈθraɪtɪs] 骨关节炎
osteochondritis	[ˌɒstɪəkɒnˈdraɪtɪs] 骨软骨炎
osteomyelitis	[ˌɒstɪəʊˌmaɪəˈlaɪtɪs] 骨髓炎
periosteomyelitis	[piəriːəʊstiːəʊmaˌɪəlaɪtɪs] 全骨炎
periostitis	[ˌperɪɒˈstaɪtɪs] 骨膜炎
spondylarthritis	[ˌspɒndɪlɑːˈθraɪtɪs] 脊椎关节炎
spondylitis	[ˌspɒndɪˈlaɪtɪs] 脊椎炎
synovitis	[ˌsaɪnəʊˈvaɪtɪs] 滑膜炎
osseous tuberculosis	[ˈɒsɪəs] [tjuːˌbɜːkjuˈləʊsɪs] 骨与关节结核

2. 骨折的类型

表 1-2-8　表示骨折类型的术语表

骨折类型	中文释义
closed fracture	闭合性骨折
Colles' fracture	桡骨下端骨折
comminuted fracture	粉碎性骨折
complete fracture	完全性骨折
compound fracture	有创骨折
double fracture	双骨折
greenstick fracture	青枝骨折
impacted fracture	嵌入骨折
incomplete fracture	不完全骨折
splintered fracture	粉碎性骨折

3. 骨骼系统病理术语

表 1-2-9　骨骼系统病理术语表

骨骼系统病理术语	中文释义
achondroplasia	[eɪˌkɒndrəˈpleɪzɪə] 软骨发育不全
acrocephaly	[ˌækrəʊˈsefəlɪ] 尖头
acromegaly	[ˌækrəʊˈmegəlɪ] 肢端肥大症
amelia	[əˈmiːljə] 无肢
anencephalia	[eɪnɪnkeˈfəlɪə] 无脑症
ankylosis	[ˌæŋkɪˈləʊsɪs] 关节僵硬
arthralgia	[ɑːˈθrældʒə] 关节痛
arthrocele	[ɑːθˈrəʊseliː] 关节肿大
arthropathy	[ɑːθrɔpəθɪ] 关节病
arthrosclerosis	[ɑːθrɒsklərəʊsɪs] 关节硬化
chondroblastoma	[kɒndrɒbˈlɑːstəmə] 成软骨细胞瘤
chondrofibroma	[kɒndrɒfaɪbˈrəʊmə] 软骨纤维瘤
chondroma	[kɒnˈdrəʊmə] 软骨瘤
chondromalacia	[kɒndrəʊməˈleɪʃə] 软骨软化
chondromyoma	[kɒndrəʊmaɪˈəʊmə] 软骨肌瘤
chondronecrosis	[tʃɒndrəʊnekˈrəʊsɪs] 软骨坏死
chondrosarcoma	[ˌkɒndrəʊsɑːˈkəʊmə] 软骨肉瘤
clubfoot	[ˈklʌbfʊt] 畸形足；弯脚
clubhand	[ˈklʌbhænd] 畸形手
coccygodynia	[kɒksɪgəʊˈdɪnɪə] coccygodynia 尾骨痛，尾痛症
coxodynia	[ˌkɒksəˈdɪnɪə] 髋关节结核
craniorachischisis	[kreɪniːəʊrætʃɪsˈkaɪsɪs] 颅脊柱裂
craniostosis	[kreɪniːəʊsˈtəʊsɪs] 颅缝骨化
dysostosis	[dɪsɒsˈtəʊsɪs] 骨发育障碍
exostosis	[ˌeksɒsˈtəʊsɪs] 外生骨疣
genu varus	膝关节外翻
giantism	[ˈdʒaɪəntɪzəm] 巨大畸形
gout	[gaʊt] 痛风
hemarthrosis	[ˌhemɑːˈθrəʊsɪs] 关节积血

续表

骨骼系统病理术语	中文释义
hydrarthrosis	[ˌhaɪdrɑːˈθrəʊsɪs] 关节积水
kyphosis	[kaɪˈfəʊsɪs] 驼背
lordosis	[lɔːˈdəʊsɪs] 脊柱前弯症
lumbago	[lʌmˈbeɪɡəʊ] 腰痛
macrobrachia	[mækrəʊˈbrækjə] 巨臂
macrognathia	[mækrɒɡˈnæθɪə] 巨颌
macropodia	[məkrɒˈpəʊdɪə] 巨足
opisthognathism	[ɒpɪsˈθɒɡnəθɪzm] 后退颌；颌后缩
ostealgia	[ˌɒstɪˈældʒɪə] 骨痛
osteoblastoma	[ˌɒstɪəʊblæsˈtəʊmə] 成骨细胞瘤
osteodystrophy	[ˌɒstɪəʊˈdɪstrəfɪ] 骨营养不良；骨营养障碍
osteoma	[ˌɒstɪˈəʊmə] 骨瘤；脑壳瘤
osteomalacia	[ˌɒstɪəʊməˈleɪʃɪə] 骨软化；软骨病
osteonecrosis	[ɒstɪəʊneˈkrəʊsɪs] 骨坏死
osteopathy	[ˌɒstɪˈɒpəθɪ] 骨病；整骨疗法
osteopetrosis	[ˌɒstɪəʊpɪˈtrəʊsɪs] 骨硬化病
osteopoikilosis	[ɒstɪəʊpɔɪkɪˈləʊsɪs] 脆弱性骨硬化
osteosarcoma	[ˌɒstɪəʊsɑːˈkəʊmə] 骨肉瘤
osteosclerosis	[ˌɒstɪəʊsklɪəˈrəʊsɪs] 骨硬化
prognathism	[prɒɡˈneɪθɪzəm] 凸颚；凸颌
rickets	[ˈrɪkɪts] 佝偻病
scaphocephaly	[ˌskæfəʊˈsefəlɪ] 舟状头
scoliosis	[ˌskəʊlɪˈəʊsɪs] 脊柱侧凸
syndactylia	[sɪnˈdæktɪlɪə] 并指；并趾；合指征

（三）骨骼系统检查术语

表 1-2-10　骨骼系统检查术语表

骨骼系统检查术语	中文释义
arthrectomy	[ɑːθrektəmɪ] 关节切除术
arthrocentesis	[ˌɑːθrəʊsenˈtiːsɪs] 关节穿刺术

续表

骨骼系统检查术语	中文释义
arthrodesis	[ɑːˈθrɒdəsɪs] 关节固定术
arthrography	[ɑːθrɒgrəfɪ] 关节摄影术
arthroplasty	[ˌɑːθrəʊˈplæstɪ] 关节成形术
arthroscopy	[ɑːˈθrɒskəpɪ] 关节镜检查
arthrotomy	[ɑːθrɒtəmɪ] 关节切开术
bursectomy	[bəˈsektəmɪ] 黏液囊切除术
bursotomy	[ˈbɜːsətəmɪ] 黏液囊切开术
carpectomy	[kɑːˈpektəmɪ] 腕骨切除术
chondrectomy	[kɒnˈdrektəmɪ] 软骨切除术
chondrotomy	[ˈkɒndrəʊtəmɪ] 软骨切开术
clavicotomy	[kˈlævɪkətəmɪ] 锁骨切断术
laminectomy	[ˌlæmɪˈnektəmɪ] 椎板切除术
lumbar puncture	腰椎穿刺
ostectomy	[ɒˈstektəmɪ] 骨切开术
osteoclasis	[ˌɒstɪˈɒkləsɪs] 骨破折
osteoplasty	[ˈɒstɪəplæstɪ] 骨成形术
osteorrhaphy	[ɒsˈtɔːrəfɪ] 骨缝合术
osteotomy	[ˌɒstɪˈɒtəmɪ] 截骨术，骨切开术
pubiotomy	[pjuːbɪˈɒtəmɪ] 耻骨切开术
scapulopexy	[skæpjʊləˈpeksɪ] 肩胛固定术
sternotomy	[stəːˈnɒtəmɪ] 胸骨切开术

（四）骨骼系统药学术语

表 1-2-11　骨骼系统药学术语表

骨骼系统药学术语	中文释义
NSAID（*nonsteroidal anti-inflammatory drug*）	非甾体抗炎药
corticosteroid	[ˌkɔːtɪkəʊˈstɪərɒɪd] 皮质类固醇；皮质甾（类）
gold therapy	金疗法

三、肌肉系统

(一) 肌肉系统词根和组合形式

表 1-2-12 肌肉系统词根和组合形式表

词根和组合形式	举例
brachi/o-（branch, arm）	*brachio*cephalic [breɪtʃiːəʊˈkefælɪk] 头臂动脉的
cephal/o-（head）	*cephalo*cele [ˈsefələʊsiːl] 脑膨出
cervic/o-（neck）	*cervico*thoracic [sɜːvɪkəʊθəˈræsɪk] 颈胸的
fasci/o-（fascia）	*fascio*plasty [fæʃɪəˈplæstɪ] 筋膜成形术
leio-（smooth）	*leio*dystonia [laɪəʊdɪsˈtəʊnɪə] 平滑肌张力障碍
muscul/o-（muscle）	*musculo*skeletal [ˌmʌskjʊləʊˈskelətəl] 骨骼的
tend/o-, tendin/o-（tendon）	*tendino*plasty [tendɪˈnɒplæstɪ] 腱成形术 *tendi*nitis [ˌtendɪˈnaɪtɪs] 腱炎

(二) 肌肉系统临床和病理

1. 肌肉系统炎症和感染术语

表 1-2-13 肌肉系统炎症和感染术语表

肌肉系统炎症和感染术语	中文释义
dermatomyositis	[ˈdəmətəʊˌmaɪəˈsaɪtɪs] 皮肌炎
fasciitis	[ˌfæsɪˈaɪtɪs] 筋膜炎
fibromyitis	[faɪbrəʊmɪˈaɪtɪs] 纤维性肌炎
myocellulitis	[maɪəseljʊˈlaɪtɪs] 肌蜂窝织炎
myofascitis	[maɪəʊfæˈsaɪtɪs] 腰背肌损伤
myositis	[ˌmaɪəʊˈsaɪtɪs] 肌炎
myotenositis	[maɪəˈtenəsaɪtɪs] 肌腱炎
tenositis	[tenəˈsaɪtɪs] 腱炎
tenosynovitis	[tenəʊsɪnəˈvaɪtɪs] 腱鞘炎

2. 肌肉系统病理术语

表 1-2-14 肌肉系统病理术语表

肌肉系统病理术语	中文释义
amyoplasia	[eɪmaɪəpˈleɪzɪə] 肌发育不全

续表

肌肉系统病理术语	中文释义
amyotonia	[ˌeɪˌmaɪəˈtəʊnɪə] 肌张力缺失，肌弛缓
amyotrophy	[ˌeɪmaɪˈɒtrəfɪ] 肌萎缩
dystonia	[dɪsˈtəʊnɪə] 肌张力障碍
leiomyoma	[laɪəʊmaɪˈəʊmə] 平滑肌瘤
leiomyosarcoma	[ˈlaɪəʊˌmaɪəʊsɑːˈkəʊmə] 平滑肌肉瘤
myasthenia gravis	[ˈgrɑːvɪs, ˈgræ-, ˈgreɪ-] 重症肌无力
myoblastoma	[maɪəʊblæsˈtəʊmə] 成肌细胞瘤
myodystrophy	[maɪəʊˈdɪstrəfɪ] 肌营养不良
myofibrosis	[maɪɔːfaɪbˈrəʊsɪs] 肌纤维变性
myoma	[maɪˈəʊmə] 肌瘤
myoparalysis	[ˈmaɪəʊpərələsɪs] 肌瘫痪
myotonia	[ˌmaɪəˈtəʊnɪə] 肌强直
myalgia	[maɪˈældʒə] 肌痛
myoclonus	[maɪˈɒklənəs] 肌阵挛
myodystonia	[maɪɒˈdɪstnjə] 肌张力障碍
myolysis	[ˌmaɪəʊˈlaɪsɪs] 肌溶解；肌肉分解
myomalacia	[ˌmaɪəʊməˈlæsɪə] 肌软化
myonecrosis	[maɪɒˈnekrəʊsɪs] 肌坏死
myopathy	[maɪˈɒpəθɪ] 肌病
myosclerosis	[maɪɒsklɪəˈrəʊsɪs] 肌硬化症
myospasm	[maɪɒsˈpæzəm] 肌痉挛
tenodynia	[ˈtenədɪnɪə] 腱痛
tetany	[ˈtetənɪ] 手足抽搐；强直
tic	[tɪk] 抽搐

（三）肌肉系统检查术语

表 1-2-15 肌肉系统检查术语表

肌肉系统检查术语	中文释义
electromyography	[ɪˌlektrəʊmaɪˈɒgrəfɪ] 肌电图学
fasciectomy	[fəˈsɪəktəmɪ] 筋膜切除术
fascioplasty	[fæʃɪəˈplæstɪ] 筋膜成形术

续表

肌肉系统检查术语	中文释义
fasciorrhaphy	[ˈfæʃɪərəfɪ] 筋膜缝术
myectomy	[maɪˈektəmɪ] 肌切除术
myoglobin	[ˌmaɪəʊˈgləʊbɪn] 肌红蛋白
myokinesimeter	[maɪəʊkɪnɪˈsɪmɪtə] 肌收缩力计
myoplasty	[ˈmaɪəplæstɪ] 肌整形术
myorrhaphy	[maɪˈɒrəfɪ] 肌缝合术
myotenotomy	[maɪəˈtenəʊtəmɪ] 肌腱切断术
myotomy	[maɪˈɒtəmɪ] 肌切开术
tenodesis	[teˈnəʊdiːsɪs] 腱固定术
tenoplasty	[tenəpˈlæstɪ] 腱成形术
tenorrhaphy	[tɪˈnɒrəfɪ] 腱缝合术；缝腱术
tenotomy	[eˈnɒtəmɪ] 腱切断术；割腱术

（四）肌肉系统药学术语

表 1-2-16　肌肉系统药学术语表

肌肉系统药学术语	中文释义
Muscle relaxant	肌肉松弛剂
antispasmodic	[ˌæntɪspæzˈmɒdɪk] 止痉挛的

四、循环系统

（一）循环系统词根和组合形式

表 1-2-17　循环系统词根和组合形式术语表

循环系统词根和组合形式	举例
aort/o-（the great artery, aorta）	*aort*itis [eəˈtaɪtɪs] 主动脉炎，织脉炎，
arteriol/o-（little artery）	*arteriol*opathy [ɑːtɪəˈraɪələpæθɪ] 小动脉病
ather/o-（fatty deposit, fatty degeneration）	*athero*sclerosis [ˌæθərəʊsklɪˈrəʊsɪs] 动脉粥样硬化
atri/o-（atrium）	*atrio*septopexy [ˈɑːtriːəʊseptɒpeksɪ] 房间隔修补术
coron/o-（crown, heart）	*coron*ary [ˈkɒrənrɪ] 冠状动脉或静脉的
embol/o-（embolus, plug）	*embol*ectomy [ˌembəˈlektəmɪ] 栓子切除术

续表

循环系统词根和组合形式	举例
eosin/o-（red, rosy, dawn-colored）	*eosino*phil [ˌiːəˈsɪnəfɪl] 嗜曙红细胞
hem/o-（blood）	*hemo*rrhage [ˈhemərɪdʒ] 出血；溢血
hemangi/o-（blood vessel）	*hemangi*oma [hiːˌmændʒiːˈəʊmə] 血管瘤
kary/o-（nucleus）	mega*karyo*cyte [megəˈkærɪəʊsaɪt] 巨核细胞
phleb/o-（blood vessel, vein）	*phleb*itis [fləˈbaɪtɪs] 静脉炎
sanguin-（blood）	*sangui*ferous [sæŋˈgwɪfərəs] 含血的
ser/o-（serum）	*sero*diagnosis [sɪərəʊdaɪəgˈnəʊsɪs] 血清诊断
sphygm/o-（pulse）	*sphygmo*meter [sfɪgˈmɒmɪtə] 脉波记
steth/o-（chest）	*stetho*scope [ˈsteθəskəʊp] 听诊器
thromb/o-（clot）	*thrombo*angiitis [θrɒmbəʊændʒɪˈaɪtɪs] 血栓血管炎
valvul/o-（valvule）	*valvul*itis [ˌvælvjʊˈlaɪtɪs] 心瓣炎
vas/o-（vessel, duct）	*vaso*constriction [ˌveɪzəʊkənˈstrɪkʃn] 血管收缩
ven/i-, ven/o-（vein）	*veno*gram [ˈvenəgræm] 静脉造影
ventricul/o-（ventricle）	*ventriculo*tomy [ventrɪkjʊˈlɒtəʊmɪ] 心室切开术
-tension（tension）	hyper*tension* [ˌhaɪpəˈtenʃn] 高血压
-version（turning）	cardio*version* [kɑːdɪəˈvɜːʃən] 心律转变法

（二）循环系统临床和病理术语

1. 循环系统炎症和感染术语表

表 1-2-18　循环系统炎症和感染术语表

循环系统炎症和感染术语	中文释义
arteritis	[ˌɑːtəˈraɪtɪs] 动脉炎
bacteremia	[bæktəˈrɪmɪə] 菌血症
carditis	[kɑːˈdaɪtɪs] 心脏炎
endarteritis	[ˌendɑːtəˈraɪtɪs] 动脉内膜炎
endocarditis	[ˌendəʊkɑːˈdaɪtɪs] 心内膜炎
leukocyte	[ˈluːkəsaɪts] 白细胞
lymphadenitis	[lɪmˌfædɪˈnaɪtɪs] 淋巴腺炎
myocarditis	[ˌmaɪəʊkɑːˈdaɪtɪs] 心肌炎
panarteritis	[pænɑːtəˈraɪtɪs] 全身动脉炎
periarteritis	[ˌperɪˌɑːtəˈraɪtɪs] 动脉周围炎

第一部分　医学英语

续表

循环系统炎症和感染术语	中文释义
phlebitis	[fləˈbaɪtɪs] 静脉炎
polyarteritis	[ˈpɒlɪˌɑːtəˈraɪtɪs] 多动脉炎
septicemia	[ˌseptɪˈsiːmɪə] 败血症；败血病
splenitis	[splɪˈnaɪtɪs] 脾炎
thromboangiitis	[ˌθrɒmbəʊˌændʒɪˈaɪtɪs] 血栓血管炎；血栓脉管炎
thrombophlebitis	[ˌθrɒmbəʊflɪˈbaɪtɪs] 血栓性静脉炎

2. 循环系统出血术语

表1-2-19　循环系统出血表达术语表

循环系统出血术语	中文释义
epistaxis	[ˌepɪˈstæksɪs] 鼻出血
hematencephalon	[hiːmætenˈsefələn] 脑出血
hematocele	[ˈhemətəʊsiːl] 囊内积血
hematoma	[ˌheməˈtəʊmə] 血肿
hematomphalocele	[hiːmætɒmˈfæləsiːl] 血脐疝
hematopericardium	[hemætəʊperɪˈkɑːdjəm] 心包积血
hematorrhea	[hiːmətəʊˈriːə] 大出血
hemophthalmia	[hiːmɒfˈθælmɪə] 眼球积血
melena	[məˈliːnə] 黑便
menorrhagia	[ˌmenəˈreɪdʒɪə] 月经过多

3. 循环系统血液病理术语

表1-2-20　循环系统血液病理表达术语表

循环系统血液病理术语	中文释义
agranulocytosis	[eɪˌgrænjələsaɪˈtəʊsɪs] 粒性白细胞缺乏症
anemia	[əˈniːmɪə] 贫血症
hemophilia	[ˌhiːməˈfɪlɪə] 血友病
leukemia	[luːˈkiːmɪə] 白血病
polycythemia	[pɒlɪsaɪˈθiːmjə] 红细胞增多症
sickle cell anemia	镰状细胞性贫血

4. 循环系统病理术语

表 1-2-21　循环系统病理表达术语表

循环系统病理术语	中文释义
aneurysm	[ˈænjərɪzəm] 动脉瘤
angialgia	[ˈændʒɪəldʒə] 血管痛
angina	[ænˈdʒaɪnə] 心绞痛
angina pectoris	[ænˌdʒaɪnəˈpektərɪs] 心绞痛
angiosclerosis	[ændʒiːəʊskləˈrəʊsɪs] 血管硬化
angiostenosis	[eɪndʒiːəʊsteˈnəʊsɪs] 血管狭窄
arrhythmia	[əˈrɪθmɪə] 心律不齐
arteriomalacia	[ɑːtɪəərɪəməˈleɪʃə] 动脉软化
atherosclerosis	[ˌæθərəʊsklɪˈrəʊsɪs] 动脉硬化
bradycardia	[brædɪˈkɑːdɪə] 心搏徐缓
cardiac arrest	心搏停止
cardiac hypertrophy	心脏肥大
cardiac murmur	心脏杂音
cardialgia	[ˌkɑːdɪˈældʒɪə] 心灼痛
cardiomegaly	[kɑːdɪəʊˈmegəlɪ] 心脏扩大症
cardionecrosis	[kɑːdaɪənekˈrəʊsɪs] 心坏死
cardioptosis	[kɑːdaɪɒpˈtəʊsɪs] 心脏下垂
congestive heart failure	充血性心力衰竭
cor pulmonale	[ˈkɔːˌpuməˈnælɪ] 肺心病
cyanosis	[ˌsaɪəˈnəʊsɪs] 发绀
dextrocardia	[ˌdekstrəʊˈkɑːdɪə] 右位心
embolism	[ˈembəlɪzəm] 血栓
erythremia	[erɪˈθriːmɪə] 红细胞增多（症）
erythrocytosis	[ɪrɪθrəʊsaɪˈtəʊsɪs] 红细胞增多（症）
erythropenia	[ɪrɪθrəˈpiːnɪə] 红细胞减少
fibrillation	[ˌfɪbrɪˈleɪʃən] 纤维性颤动
granulocytopenia	[grænjʊləsaɪtəˈpiːnɪə] 粒细胞减少
granulocytosis	[grænjʊləʊsaɪˈtəʊsɪs] 粒细胞增多
heart block	心传导阻滞

续表

循环系统病理术语	中文释义
hemangiectasis	[hiːmændʒɪˈektəsɪs] 血管扩张
hematocytopenia	[hemætəsiːtəʊˈpiːnɪə] 血细胞减少
hemoglobinemia	[hiːməgləʊbɪˈniːmɪə] 血红蛋白血症
Hodgkin's disease	[ˈhɒdʒkɪn] 淋巴瘤
hypertension	[ˌhaɪpəˈtenʃn] 高血压；过度紧张
hypotension	[ˌhaɪpəʊˈtenʃən] 低血压
infarct	[ɪnˈfɑːkt] 梗死
ischemia	[ɪsˈkiːmɪə] 局部贫血
leukopenia	[ˌluːkəˈpiːnɪə] 白血球减少症
lymphadenopathy	[lɪmˌfædəˈnɒpəθɪ] 淋巴结病
lymphedema	[lɪmfɪˈdiːmə] 淋巴水肿
lymphocytosis	[ˌlɪmfəʊsaɪˈtəʊsɪs] 淋巴球增多
lymphoma	[lɪmˈfəʊmə] 淋巴瘤
monocytopenia	[mɒnəʊsaɪtəˈpiːnɪə] 单核细胞减少症
monocytosis	[mɒnəʊsaɪˈtəʊsɪs] 单核细胞增多（症）
neutropenia	[ˌnjuːtrəˈpiːnɪə] 嗜中性白血球减少症
occlusion	[əˈkluːʒn] 闭塞；梗死
palpitation	[ˌpælpɪˈteɪʃn] 悸动
phlebangioma	[flɪbændʒɪˈəʊmə] 静脉瘤
phlebosclerosis	[flebəʊsklɪəˈrəʊsɪs] 慢性静脉炎；静脉硬化
phlebostenosis	[flɪbɒsteˈnəʊsɪs] 静脉狭窄
polyemia	[pɒlɪˈiːmɪə] 多血（症）
pulmonary stenosis	肺动脉瓣狭窄
reticulocytopenia	[rɪtɪkjʊləsaɪtəʊˈpiːnɪə] 网状细胞减少
tetralogy of fallot	法洛四联症
thrombus	[ˈθrɒmbəs] 血栓
varicose	[ˈværɪkəʊs] 静脉曲张的
vasoconstriction	[ˌveɪzəʊkənˈstrɪkʃn] 血管收缩
vasodilation	[ˌveɪzəʊdaɪˈleɪʃn] 血管舒张
vasospasm	[ˈveɪsəʊspæzm] 血管痉挛

（三）循环系统检查术语

表 1-2-22　循环系统检查表达术语表

循环系统检查术语	中文释义
Activated partial thromboplastin time	活化部分凝血激酶时间
anastomosis	[ənæstəˈməʊsɪs] 吻合术；接合
aneurysmectomy	[ænjʊərɪzˈmektəmɪ] 动脉瘤切除术
aneurysmoplasty	[ænjʊərɪzˈmɒplæstɪ] 动脉瘤成形术
aneurysmotomy	[ænjʊərɪzˈməʊtəmɪ] 动脉瘤切开术
angiectomy	[ændˈʒiːktəmɪ] 血管切除术
angiocardiogram	[ændʒiːəʊˈkɑːdɪəʊgræm] 心血管照片
angiogram	[ˈɑnjɪəˈgram] 血管造影片
angioneurectomy	[ændʒənjʊəˈrektəmɪ] 血管神经切除术
angiorrhaphy	[ˈændʒɪrəfɪ] 血管缝术，血管修补术
angiostomy	[ˈeɪndʒiːəʊstəmɪ] 血管造口术，血管吻合术
aortotomy	[eəˈtəʊtəmɪ] 主动脉切开术
arterioplasty	[ɑːtɪəraɪɒpˈlæstɪ] 动脉成形术
arteriorrhaphy	[ˈɑːtɪərɪərəfɪ] 动脉缝术，动脉修补术
arteriotomy	[ˈɑːtɪərɪətəmɪ] 动脉切开术
artificial cardiac pacemaker	人工心脏起搏器
atriotomy	[ˈɑːtrɪətəmɪ] 心房切开术
ballistocardiogram	[bəlɪstəˈkɑːdɪəʊgræm] 心冲击描记图
blood culture	血培养
bone marrow aspiration	骨髓穿刺
cardiac catheterization	心导管插入
cardiocentesis	[kɑːdɪəsenˈtiːsɪs] 心脏穿刺术
cardiotomy	[kɑːdɪˈɒtəmɪ] 心切开术；贲门切开术
coagulation tests	凝血试验
complete blood count（CBC）	全细胞计数
coronary artery bypass graft（CABG）	冠状动脉旁路移植术
differential blood count	血细胞分类技术
echocardiography	[ekəʊkɑːdɪˈɒgrəfɪ] 超声波心动描记术

第一部分　医学英语

续表

循环系统检查术语	中文释义
electrocardiogram（ECG/EKG）	[ɪˌlektrəʊˈkɑːdɪəʊgræm] 心电图
embolectomy	[ˌembəˈlektəmɪ] 栓子切除术
erythrocyte sedimentation rate	红细胞沉降率
exercise stress test	运动负荷试验
heart transplantation	心脏移植
hematocrit	[ˈhemətəʊkrɪt] 血球比容计；血球密度
hemogram	[ˈhiːməgræm] 血像；血图
hemolysis	[hɪˈmɒlɪsɪs] 溶血
hemorrhoidectomy	[ˌhemərɔɪˈdektəmɪ] 痔切除术
lymphadenectomy	[lɪmfədˈnektəmɪ] 淋巴结切除术
lymphangiectomy	[lɪmpˈhædʒɪːktəmɪ] 淋巴管切除术
Open heart surgery	心脏直视手术
percutaneous transluminal coronary angioplasty（PTCA）	经皮腔内冠状动脉成形术
pericardiocentesis	[ˈperɪkɑːdɪəʊsenˈtiːsɪs] 心包（放液）穿刺术
phlebophlebostomy	[flɪbəflɪˈbɒstəmɪ] 静脉吻合术
phleboplasty	[flɪˈbəʊpləstɪ] 静脉成形术
phleborrhaphy	[flɪˈbɒrəfɪ] 静脉缝术
Prothrombin time	前凝血酶时间，凝血酶原时间
Serum enzyme tests	血清酶测试
splenectomy	[splɪˈnektəmɪ] 脾切除术
splenopexy	[ˈspliːnəˌpeksɪ] 脾固定术
splenotomy	[splɪˈnɒtəmɪ] 脾切开术
thrombectomy	[θrɒmˈbektəmɪ] 血栓切除术
thrombolysis	[θˈrɒmbəʊlɪsɪs] 血栓溶解
thymectomy	[θaɪˈmektəmɪ] 胸腺切除术
valvuloplasty	[vælvjʊˈləplæstɪ] 瓣膜成形术
valvulotomy	[vælvjʊˈlɒtəmɪ] 瓣膜切开术
venipuncture	[ˈveniˌpʌŋktʃə] 静脉穿刺的；静脉针灸
ventriculotomy	[ventrɪkjʊˈləʊtəʊmɪ] 心室切开术

（四）循环系统药学术语

表 1-2-23　循环系统药学表达术语表

循环系统药学术语	中文释义
anticoagulant	[ˌæntɪkəʊˈæɡjələnt] 抗凝的
fibrinolytic	[ˌfaɪbrɪnəʊˈlaɪsɪs] 纤维蛋白溶解
hemostatic	[ˌhiːməˈstætɪk] 止血的
antihypertensive	[ˈænti:hɑɪpəˈtensɪv] 抗高血压的；降压的
diuretic	[ˌdaɪjuˈretɪk] 利尿剂
β-adrenergic blocking agent（β-blocker）	β 类肾上腺素阻断剂
calcium channel blocker	钙离子通道
inotropic	[ˌiːnəˈtrɒpɪk] 影响肌肉收缩力的
cardiotonic	[kɑːdɪəʊˈtɒnɪk] 强心的
vasodilator	[ˌvæsəʊdaɪˈleɪtə] 血管舒张药
antianginal	[ænˈtiːəŋɪnl] 防心绞痛的，减轻心绞痛的

五、呼吸系统

（一）呼吸系统词根和组合形式

表 1-2-24　呼吸系统词根和组合形式术语表

呼吸系统词根和组合形式	举例
adenoid/o-（adenoid）	*adenoid*ectomy [ˌædɪnɒɪˈdektəmɪ] 增殖腺切除术
alvel/o-（alveous）	*alve*olar [ælˈviːələ(r)] 齿槽的；肺胞的；胞状的
anthrac/o-（charcoal）	*anthrac*osis [ænθrəˈkəʊsɪs] 硅肺病
atel/o-（incomplete, imperfect）	*atel*ectasis [ˌætəˈlektəsɪs] 肺膨胀不全
bronch/o-（bronchus）	*bronch*iole [ˈbrɒŋkɪəʊl] 细支气管
coni/o-（dust）	pneumo*coni*osis[ˌnjuːməkəʊnɪˈəʊsɪs] 肺尘病
epiglott/o-（epiglottis）	*epiglott*idectomy[epɪɡlɒtɪˈdektəmɪ] 会厌切除术
lob/o-（lobe）	*lob*ectomy [ləʊˈbektəmɪ] 叶切除术
nas/o-（nose）	*nas*ogastric [neɪzəʊˈɡæstrɪk] 鼻胃的
oxy-（oxygen）	*oxy*genate [ˈɒksɪdʒəneɪt] 氧化
pector/o-（chest）	*pector*algia [pektəˈrældʒə] 胸痛

续表

呼吸系统词根和组合形式	举例
pharyng/o-（pharygn）	*pharyng*oplegia [fərɪŋgəˈpledʒɪə] 咽肌麻痹
phren/o-（diaphragm）	*phren*ospasm [frenəˈspæzm] 膈痉挛
pneumat/o-（air, breath）	*pneumat*ocardia [nju:mætəˈkɑ:dɪə] 心积气，心腔积气
pneumon/o-（lung, air）	*pneumon*ectomy [ˌnju:məˈnektəmɪ] 肺切除术
pulmon/o-（lung, air）	*pulmo*lith [pʌlˈməʊlɪθ] 肺石
spir/o-（breathe）	*spiro*meter [ˌspaɪəˈrɒmɪtə] 肺活量计
tonsil/o-（tonsils）	*tonsil*litis [ˌtɒnsəˈlaɪtɪs] 扁桃体炎
trache/o-（trachea）	*trache*itis [ˌtreɪkɪˈaɪtɪs] 气管炎
-capnia（carbon dioxide）	hyper*capnia* [ˌhaɪpəˈkæpnɪə] 血碳酸过多症
-phonia（voice）	dys*phonia* [dɪsˈfəʊnɪə] 发声困难；言语障碍
-ptysis（spitting）	hemo*ptysis* [hɪˈmɒptəsɪs] 咯血，咳血
-pnea（breathe）	a*pnea* [ˈæpnɪə] 呼吸暂停；室息
-thorax（chest）	Pneumo*thorax* [ˌnju:məˈθɔ:ræks] 气胸

（二）呼吸系统临床和病理术语

1. 呼吸系统炎症和感染术语

表 1-2-25 呼吸系统炎症和感染术语表

呼吸系统临床术语	中文释义
arytenoiditis	[ærɪti:nɒɪˈdaɪtɪs] 杓状软骨炎
bronchiolitis	[ˌbrɒŋkɪəʊˈlaɪtɪs] 细支气管炎
bronchitis	[brɒŋˈkaɪtɪs] 支气管炎
bronchopneumonia	[brɒntʃɒpnju:ˈməʊnjə] 毛细支气管炎
bronchosinusitis	[brɒntʃəʊzɪˈnəsaɪtɪs] 支气管鼻窦炎
chorditis	[kɔ:ˈdaɪtɪs] 声带炎
diphtheria	[dɪfˈθɪərɪə] 白喉
epiglottitis	[epɪglɒˈtaɪtɪs] 会厌炎
histoplasmosis	[hɪstəʊplæzˈməʊsɪs] 网状内皮细胞真菌病
influenza	[ˌɪnfluˈenzə] 流行性感冒
laryngitis	[ˌlærɪnˈdʒaɪtɪs] 喉炎
laryngopharyngitis	[lærɪŋgəʊfærɪɒpədˈʒaɪtɪs] 喉咽炎
laryngotracheitis	[lərɪŋgəʊtrækɪˈaɪtɪs] 喉气管炎

续表

呼吸系统临床术语	中文释义
laryngotracheobronchitis	[ləriŋgəutreikiəbrɒnˈkaitis] 喉气管支气管炎
mediastinitis	[mediəsˈtinaitəs] 纵隔炎
nasopharyngitis	[ˌneizəuˌfærənˈdʒaitis] 鼻咽炎
pansinusitis	[pænsainəˈsaitis] 全窦炎
pertussis	[pəˈtʌsis] 百日咳
pharyngitis	[ˌfærinˈdʒaitis] 咽炎
pharyngorhinitis	[færiŋgɔːˈhinaitəs] 咽鼻炎
pharyngolaryngitis	[færiŋgəulərindˈʒaitis] 咽喉炎
pleurisy	[ˈpluərəsi] 肋膜炎；胸膜炎
pleuropericarditis	[pluərəperikɑːˈdaitis] 胸膜心包炎
pleuropneumonia	[ˈpluərəunjuː(ː)ˈməunjə] 肋膜肺炎
pneumonia	[njuːˈməuniə] 肺炎
rhinitis	[raiˈnaitis] 鼻炎
rhinolaryngitis	[rinəulərindˈʒaitis] 鼻喉炎
rhinitis	[raiˈnaitis] 鼻炎
rhinolaryngitis	[rinəulərindˈʒaitis] 鼻喉炎
rhinopharyngitis	[rainəufærinˈdʒaitis] 鼻咽炎
sinusitis	[ˌsainəˈsaitis] 窦炎
tracheitis	[ˌtreikiˈaitis] 气管炎
tracheobronchitis	[treikiəbrɒŋˈkaitis] 气管支气管炎
tuberculosis	[tjuːˌbɜːkjuˈləusis] 肺结核

2. 呼吸系统病理术语

表 1-2-26 呼吸系统病理表达术语表

呼吸系统病理术语	中文释义
anoxemia	[ənɒkˈsiːmiə] 血液缺氧症
anoxia	[æˈnɒksiə] 缺氧症
aphonia	[æˈfəunjə] 失声；无声；失音症
apnea	[ˈæpniə] 呼吸暂停；窒息
asphyxia	[æsˈfiksiə] 窒息
asthma	[ˈæsmə] 哮喘
atelectasis	[ˌætəˈlektəsis] 肺膨胀不全

续表

呼吸系统病理术语	中文释义
bradypnea	[bˈreɪdɪpnɪə] 呼吸徐缓，呼吸过慢
bronchial adenoma	支气管腺瘤
bronchiectasis	[brɑŋkɪˈektəsɪs] 支气管扩张；支气管扩张症
broncholithiasis	[brɒnkəlɪˈθaɪəsɪs] 支气管石病，支气管结石
bronchoplegia	[brɒntʃəpˈliːdʒə] 支气管麻痹
bronchorrhea	[brɒnˈkɒriː] 支气管黏液溢
bronchospasm	[ˈbrɒŋkəˌspæzəm] 支气管痉挛
bronchostenosis	[brɒntʃəʊseˈnəʊsɪs] 支气管狭窄
cheyne-stroke respiration	切斯氏呼吸
chronic obstructive pulmonary disease（COPD）	慢性阻塞性肺疾病
croup	[kruːp] 哮吼咳嗽
cystic fibrosis	[ˌsɪstɪkfaɪˈbrəʊsɪs] 囊性纤维变性
deviated septum of nose	鼻中隔偏曲
dysphonia	[dɪsˈfəʊnɪə] 发声困难；言语障碍
dyspnea	[dɪsˈpniː ə] 呼吸困难
emphysema	[ˌemfɪˈsiːmə] 肺气肿
hemopneumothorax	[hiːmɒpnjuːməʊˈθɔːræks] 血气胸
hemoptysis	[hɪˈmɒptəsɪs] 咯血，咳血
hemothorax	[ˌhiːməˈθɔːræks] 血胸；胸膜腔积血
hiccup	[ˈhɪkʌp] 打嗝
hyaline membrane disease	肺透明膜病
hydropneumothorax	[haɪdrənjuːməˈθɔːræks] 水气胸
hydrothorax	[ˌhaɪdrəˈθəʊræks] 胸膜积水
hyperpnea	[ˌhaɪpəpˈniː ə] 呼吸过度；喘息
hyperventilation	[ˌhaɪpəˌventɪˈleɪʃn] 换气过度；强力呼吸
hypoxemia	[ˌhaɪpɒkˈsiːmɪə] 血氧不足
hypoxia	[haɪˈpɒksɪə] 氧过少；低氧
laryngostenosis	[ləˌrɪŋgəʊstɪˈnəʊsɪs] 喉狭窄
laryngalgia	[lærɪŋˈgældʒɪə] 喉痛

续表

呼吸系统病理术语	中文释义
laryngoptosis	[lærɪŋˈgɒptəʊsɪs] 喉下垂
laryngorrhagia	[lærɪŋˈgɒrædʒə] 喉出血
laryngospasm	[lærɪŋˈgɒspæzəm] 喉痉挛，喉头痉挛，喉肌痉挛
oat cell carcinoma	燕麦细胞瘤
orthopnea	[ɔːˈθɒpnjəˌ ːc] 端坐呼吸；直立呼吸
pleuralgia	[pluəˈrældʒə] 胸膜痛
pneumoconiosis	[ˌnjuːməkəʊnɪˈəʊsɪs] 肺尘病
pneumohemothorax	[njuːməhiːməˈθɔːræks] 血气胸
pneumohydrothorax	[njuːməʊhaɪdrəʊˈθɔːræks] 气水胸
pneumolithiasis	[njuːməlɪˈθaɪəsɪs] 肺石病
pneumomalacia	[njuːməʊməˈleɪʃə] 肺软化
pneumomediastinum	[njuːməˈmiːdɪəstaɪnəm] 纵隔积气
pneumomelanosis	[njuːməmeləˈnəʊsɪs] 肺黑变病
pneumopyothorax	[njuːməpaɪəˈθɔːræks] 脓气胸
pneumorrhagia	[njuːməˈreɪdʒɪə] 肺出血
pneumothorax	[ˌnjuːməˈθɔːræksˌ] 气胸
polyp	[ˈpɒlɪp] 息肉
polyposis of nose	息肉病
pulmonary edema	肺水肿
pulmonary fibrosis	肺纤维化
pyothorax	[paɪəʊˈθɔːræks] 脓胸
rale	[ˈrɑːl] 啰音；水泡音
respiratory acidosis	呼吸性酸中毒
respiratory alkalosis	呼吸性碱中毒
rhonchus	[ˈrɒŋkəs] 干啰音；鼾音；诊音
sputum	[ˈspjuːtəm] 唾液；痰
stridor	[ˈstraɪdə] 喘鸣
tracheorrhagia	[træˈkɔːrædʒə] 气管出血
tracheostenosis	[trækiːəʊsteˈnəʊsɪs] 气管狭窄

（三）呼吸系统检查术语

表 1-2-27　呼吸系统检查表达术语表

呼吸系统检查术语	中文释义
arytenoidectomy	[ærɪtiːnɒɪˈdektəmɪ] 杓状软骨切除术
arytenoidopexy	[ærɪtiːnɒɪdəʊˈpeksɪ] 杓状软骨固定术
aspiration	[ˌæspəˈreɪʃn] 吸引术
auscultation	[ˌɔːskəlˈteɪʃn] 听诊
bronchogram	[bˈrɒnkəʊgræm] 支气管造影照片
bronchoplasty	[brɒntʃəpˈlæstɪ] 支气管成形术
bronchorrhaphy	[brɒnˈkɒrəfɪ] 支气管缝合术
bronchoscopy	[bˈrɒntʃəskəpɪ] 支气管窥镜检查
bronchostomy	[brɒntˈʃəʊstəmɪ] 支气管造口术
bronchotomy	[bˈrɒnʃəʊtəmɪ] 支气管切开术
chest X-ray	胸部 X 线
cordectomy	[kɒˈdektəmɪ] 声带切除术
cordopexy	[kɔːdəʊˈpeksɪ] 声带固定术
endoscope	[ˈendəskəʊp] 内窥镜；内诊镜
epiglottidectomy	[epɪglɒtɪˈdektəmɪ] 会厌切除术
ethmoidectomy	[eθmɒɪˈdektəmɪ] 筛房切除术
functional residual capacity	有效余气量，机能残气量
inspiratory capacity（Ic）	吸气量
intermittent positive-pressure breathing	间歇性正压呼吸
intubation	[ˈɪntjʊbeɪʃn] 插管（法）
laryngectomy	[ˌlærɪnˈdʒektəmɪ] 喉头切除术
laryngopharyngectomy	[lærɪŋgəʊfærɪŋˈgektəmɪ] 咽喉切除术，喉咽切除术
laryngoplasty	[lærɪŋˈgɒplæstɪ] 喉成形术
laryngoscopy	[ˌlærɪŋˈgɒskəpɪ] 喉镜检查
laryngostomy	[læˈrɪŋgəstəmɪ] 喉造口术
laryngotomy	[ˌlærɪŋˈgɒtəmɪ] 喉头剖开术
laryngotracheotomy	[lærɪŋgətˈrækɪɒtəmɪ] 喉气管切开术
Lung scan	肺部扫描

续表

呼吸系统检查术语	中文释义
percussion	[pəˈkʌʃn] 叩诊
phrenicotomy	[fˈrenɪkətəmɪ] 膈神经切断术
pleurocentesis	[pluəˈreɪsentɪzɪs] 胸腔穿刺术
pleurectomy	[plʊˈrektəmɪ] 胸膜（部分）切除术
thoracotomy	[ˌθɔːrəˈkɒtəmɪ] 胸廓切开术
thoracostomy	[ˌθɔːrəˈkɒstəmɪ] 胸廓造口术
pleurectomy	[plʊˈrektəmɪ] 胸膜（部分）切除术
pleuroparietopexy	[pluərəʊpɑːrɪtəʊˈpeksɪ] 胸膜胸壁固定术
pneumocentesis	[njuːməʊˈsentɪzɪs] 肺穿刺术,肺穿刺术
pneumonectomy	[ˌnjuːməˈnektəmɪ] 肺切除术
pneumonopexy	[njuːməˈnəʊpeksɪ] 肺固定术
pneumonorrhaphy	[njuːməˈnɔːrəfɪ] 肺缝术
pneumonotomy	[njuːˈmənəʊtəmɪ] 肺切开术
postural drainage	体位引流法
pulmonary function tests	肺功能测试
rhinoplasty	[ˈraɪnəˌplæstɪ] 鼻整形术
septectomy	[sepˈtektəmɪ] 鼻甲隔切除术,鼻中隔切除术
sinusotomy	[ˈsaɪnəsətəmɪ] 窦切开术
sputum culture	痰培养
thoracoplasty	[θɔːrəkəʊˈplæstɪ] 胸廓成形术
tracheorrhaphy	[træˈkɔːrəfɪ] 气管缝合术,气管缝术
throat culture	喉头拭子培养
tidal volume（Tv）	潮流气量
timed forced expiratory volume （Fev）	最大呼吸量
total lung capacity（TLC）	总肺活量
tracheoplasty	[trækiːəʊˈplæstɪ] 气管成形术
tracheostomy	[ˌtreɪkɪˈɒstəmɪ] 气管造口术
vital capacity	肺活量

（四）呼吸系统药学术语

表 1-2-28　呼吸系统药学表达术语表

呼吸系统药学术语	中文释义
antihistamine	[ˌæntɪˈhɪstəmiːn] 抗组胺剂
antitussive	[ˌæntɪˈtʌsɪv] 止咳药；镇咳药
bronchodilator	[ˌbrɒŋkəʊdaɪˈleɪtə] 支气管扩张药
decongestant	[ˌdiːkənˈdʒestənt] 解充血药
expectorant	[ɪkˈspektərənt] 除痰剂
mucolytic	[mjʊkəʊˈlɪtɪk] 黏液溶解的

六、消化系统

（一）消化系统词根和组合形式

表 1-2-29　消化系统词根和组合形式表

消化系统词根后缀和组合形式	举例
alveol/o-（hollow, socket of the teeth）	*alveolo*dental [ælˈvɪələʊdentl] 牙槽牙的
an/o-（anus）	*an*usitis [əˈnəsaɪtɪs] 肛门炎
append/o-（appendix）	*append*ectomy [ˌæpenˈdektəmɪ] 阑尾切除术
appendic/o-（appendix）	*appendic*itis [əˌpendəˈsaɪtɪs] 阑尾炎；盲肠炎
bil/i-（bile）	*bil*irubin [ˌbɪlɪˈruːbɪn] 胆红素
bucc/o-（cheek）	*bucc*olingual [ˈbʌkəʊlɪŋgwəl] 颊舌的
cec/o-（blind, blind gut）	*cec*itis [sɪˈsaɪtɪs] 盲肠炎
celi/o-（belly, abdomen）	*celi*ocentesis [siːlɪəʊsenˈtiːsɪs] 腹腔穿刺术
cement/o-（cementum）	*cement*oclasia [sɪmentəˈkleɪsɪə] 牙骨质破坏
cheil/o-（edge, lip, or brim）	*cheil*itis [kaɪˈlaɪtɪs] 唇炎
cholangi/o-（bile vessel）	*cholangi*ogram [kəʊˈlændʒɪəʊgræm] 胆管造影照片
chole-, chol/o-（bile）	*chole*cyst [ˈkɒləˌsɪst] 胆囊
cholecyst/o-（gallbladder）	*cholecyst*ectasia [kəʊlsɪsˈtekteɪzjə] 胆囊扩张
choledoch/o-（common bile duct）	*choledoch*olith [ˈkəʊldɒkəlɪθ] 胆总管石
col/o-（colon）	*col*onorrhagia [kələˈnɔːrædʒə] 结肠出血
dent/o-（tooth, teeth）	*dent*algia [denˈtældʒɪə] 齿痛

续表

消化系统词根后缀和组合形式	举例
dentin/o-（dentin）	*dentin*oblast [dentɪnəʊbˈlɑːst] 成牙质细胞
duoden/o-（twelve）	*duoden*ostomy [djuədɪˈnɒstəmɪ] 十二指肠切除术
esophag/o-（esophagus）	*esophag*oscope [iːˈsɒfəgəskəʊp] 食管镜
enter/o-（small intestine）	*enter*orrhea [entərɒˈrɪə] 腹泻
fec/o-（feces, stool）	*fec*al [ˈfiːkl] 排泄物的
gingiv/o-（gum）	*gingiv*itis [ˌdʒɪndʒɪˈvaɪtəs] 齿龈炎
gloss/o-（tongue）	*gloss*odynia [gˈlɒsɒdɪnɪə] 舌痛
gnath/o-（jaw）	*gnath*odynia [ˈnætəʊdɪnɪə] 颌痛
hern/i-（hernia）	*hern*ioplasty [ˈhɜːnɪəplæstɪ] [医] 疝根治手术
icter/o-（jaundice）	*icter*ohepatitis [ɪktərəʊhepəˈtaɪtɪs] 黄疸性肝炎
ile/o-（ileum, flank）	*ile*ocolitis [ɪlɪəʊkəˈlaɪtɪs] 回肠结肠炎
jejun/o-（jejunum）	*jejun*ostomy [dʒɪdʒuːˈnɒstəmɪ] 空肠造口术
labi/o-（lip）	*labi*oplasty [ˈleɪbɪəplæstɪ] 唇成形术
lapar/o-（flank,abdominal wall）	*lapar*ocele [ləˈpærəʊseliː] 腹疝
lien/o-（spleen）	*lien*itis [laɪəˈnaɪtɪs] 脾炎
lingu/o-（tongue）	sub*lingu*al [sʌbˈlɪŋgwəl] 舌下的；舌下腺的
lith/o-（calculus）	*lith*ogenesis [ˈlɪθəʊdʒenəsɪs] 造岩
mesenter/o-（mesentery）	*mesenter*itis [mezentɪˈraɪtɪs] 肠系膜炎
occlus/o-（a closing）	mal*occlus*ion [ˌmæləˈkluːʒən] 咬合不正
odont/o-（tooth, teeth）	*odont*olith [ˈɒdɒntəʊlɪθ] 牙垢，齿石
oment/o-（omentum）	*oment*orrhaphy [əʊmenˈtɒrəfɪ] 网膜缝术
orex/i-（appetite）	an*orex*ia [ˌænəˈreksɪə] 厌食症
or/o-（mouth）	*or*al [ˈɔːrəl] 口部的
orth/o-（straight）	*orth*odontics [ˌɔːθəˈdɒntɪks] 畸齿矫正学
peritone/o-（peritoneum）	*periton*itis [ˌperɪtəˈnaɪtɪs] 腹膜炎
pept/i-（digestion）	*pept*ic [ˈpeptɪk] 有助消化的；胃蛋白酶的
proct/o-（rectum）	*proct*oscope [ˈprɒktəskəʊp] 直肠镜
prosth/o-（an artificial substitute for a missing body part）	*prosth*odontics [prɒsθəˈdɒntɪks] 假牙修复学
pylor/o-（pylorus）	*pylor*ospasm [paɪlɔːrəˈspæzm] 幽门痉挛
polyp/o-（a morbid excrescence）	*polyp*osis [pɒlɪˈpəʊsɪs] 息肉病

续表

消化系统词根后缀和组合形式	举例
rect/o-（rectum）	*rect*opexy [rektəʊˈpeksɪ] 直肠固定术
saliv/o-（saliva）	*saliv*ary [səˈlaɪvərɪ] 唾液的
sphincter/o-（sphincter）	*sphincter*ectomy [sfɪŋktɪˈrektəmɪ] 括约肌切除术
splen/o-（spleen）	*splen*ocele [ˈspliːnəˌsiːl] 脾疝
stomat/o-（an opening）	*stomat*itis [ˌstəʊməˈtaɪtɪs] 口腔炎
sial/o-（saliva）	*sial*oangitis [sɪələʊændˈʒɪtɪs] 涎管炎
sigmoid/o-（sigmoid colon）	*sigmoid*ostomy [sɪɡmɔɪˈdɒstəmɪ] 乙状结肠造口术
-chlorhydria（hydrochloric acid）	a*chlorhydria* [ˌeɪklɔːˈhaɪdrɪə] 胃酸缺乏症
-crine（to secrete）	endo*crine* [ˈendəʊkrɪn] 内分泌的
-emesis（vomit）	hemat*emesis* [ˌhiːməˈteməsɪs] 咯血的
-prandial（pertaining to a meal）	pre*prandial* [ˌpriːˈprændɪəl] 餐前的

（二）消化系统临床和病理术语

1. 消化系统炎症和感染术语

表 1-2-30　消化系统炎症和感染术语表达术语表

消化系统炎症和感染术语	中文释义
anusitis	[əˈnəsaɪtɪs] 肛门炎
appendicitis	[əˌpendəˈsaɪtɪs] 阑尾炎；盲肠炎
ascariasis	[əskæˈrɪəsɪs] 蛔虫病
cheilitis	[kaɪˈlaɪtɪs] 唇炎
cholangiolitis	[ˈkəʊlədʒiːəʊlaɪtɪs] 胆小管炎，毛细胆管炎
cholangitis	[kəʊlænˈdʒaɪtɪs] 胆管炎；胆道炎
cholecystitis	[ˌkɒlɪsɪsˈtaɪtɪs] 胆囊炎
colitis	[kəˈlaɪtɪs] 结肠炎
cysticercosis	[sɪstɪsəˈkəʊsɪs] 囊（尾幼）虫病
diverticulitis	[ˌdaɪvətɪkjʊˈlaɪtɪs] 憩室炎
duodenitis	[ˌdjuːəʊdiːˈnaɪtɪs] 十二指肠炎
dysentery	[ˈdɪsəntrɪ] 痢疾
enteritis	[ˌentəˈraɪtəs] 肠炎
enterocolitis	[ˌentərəʊkəʊˈlaɪtɪs] 小肠结肠炎

续表

消化系统炎症和感染术语	中文释义
enterogastritis	[entərəʊgæstˈraɪtɪs] 胃肠炎
enterohepatitis	[ˈentərəʊhepəˈtaɪtɪs] 肠肝炎
esophagitis	[ɪsɒfəˈdʒaɪtɪs] 食道炎
gastritis	[gæˈstraɪtɪs] 胃炎
gastroduodenitis	[gæstrədjuːəʊˈdenaɪtɪs] 胃十二指肠炎
gastroenterocolitis	[ˈgæstrəʊentərəʊkəlaɪtɪz] 胃小肠结肠炎
gastroileitis	[gæstrəʊɪˈlɪaɪtɪz] 胃回肠炎
gingivitis	[ˌdʒɪndʒɪˈvaɪtəs] 齿龈炎
glossitis	[glɒˈsaɪtɪs] 舌炎
hepatitis	[ˌhepəˈtaɪtɪs] 肝炎
ileitis	[ˌɪlɪˈaɪtɪs] 回肠炎
ileocolitis	[ɪlɪəʊkəˈlaɪtɪs] 回肠结肠炎
jejunoileitis	[dʒiːdʒuːnɒɪˈlɪaɪtɪz] 空肠回肠炎
pancreatitis	[ˌpænkrɪəˈtaɪtɪs] 胰腺炎
parotitis	[ˌpærəˈtaɪtɪs] 腮腺炎；耳下腺炎
peritonitis	[ˌperɪtəˈnaɪtɪs] 腹膜炎
proctitis	[prɒkˈtaɪtɪs] 直肠炎
pulpitis	[ˈpʌlˈpaɪdɪs] 牙髓炎
sialadenitis	[ˈsaɪələdəˈnaɪtɪs] 涎腺炎
stomatitis	[ˌstəʊməˈtaɪtɪs] 口内炎；口腔炎
trichuriasis	[trɪkjʊˈraɪəsɪs] 鞭虫病

2. 消化系统病理术语

表 1-2-31 消化系统病理表达术语表

消化系统病理术语	中文释义
acholia	[eɪˈkəʊlɪə] 无胆汁（症）
achylia	[əˈkaɪljə] 胃液缺乏
anorexia	[ˌænəˈreksɪə] 厌食症
ascites	[æˈsaɪts] 腹水
bulimia	[buˈlɪmɪə] 贪食症；食欲过剩

第一部分 医学英语

续表

消化系统病理术语	中文释义
cachexia	[kəˈkeksɪə] 恶病质
cholelithiasis	[ˌkɒlɪlɪˈθʌɪəsɪs] 胆石症
cirrhosis	[səˈrəʊsɪs] 硬化
cleft lip	唇裂
cleft palate	腭裂
colic	[ˈkɒlɪk] 疝痛；疝气
constipation	[ˌkɒnstɪˈpeɪʃən] 便秘
diabetes mellitus	糖尿病
diarrhea	[ˌdaɪəˈrɪə] 腹泻；痢疾
diverticulosis	[daɪvətɪkjʊˈləʊsɪs] 憩室病
dyspepsia	[dɪsˈpepsɪə] 消化不良
emesis	[ˈeməsɪs] 呕吐
enterolith	[ˈentərəlɪθ] 肠石
enteroptosis	[entərɒpˈtəʊsɪs] 肠下垂
fistula	[ˈfɪstjʊlə] 瘘；瘘管
gastralgia	[gæsˈtrældʒɪə] 胃痛
gastrolith	[ˈgæstrəlɪθ] 胃石
gastroptosis	[gæstrɒpˈtəʊsɪs] 胃下垂
halitosis	[ˌhælɪˈtəʊsɪs] 口臭
hematemesis	[ˌhiːməˈteməsɪs] 吐血；咯血
hemoperitoneum	[hiːməʊperɪtəʊˈniːəm] 腹腔积血
hepatomegaly	[hepətəʊˈmegəlɪ] 肝肿大
hepatosplenomegaly	[hepətəʊspliːnəʊˈmegəlɪ] 肝脾大
hernia	[ˈhɜːnɪə] 疝气；脱肠
hyperbilirubinemia	[haɪpɜːbɪliːrʌbaɪˈniːmɪə] 胆红素血
hyperchlorhydria	[haɪpə(ː)klɔːˈhaɪdrɪə] 胃酸过多症
hypercholia	[haɪpəˈkəʊlɪə] 胆汁分泌过多
hyperglycemia	[ˌhaɪpəglaɪˈsiːmɪə] 多糖症；高血糖症
ileus	[ˈɪlɪəs] 肠闭塞
intussuception	肠套叠

续表

消化系统病理术语	中文释义
jaundice	[ˈdʒɔːndɪs] 黄疸
leukoplakia	[luːkəˈpleɪkɪə] 黏膜白斑病
macroglossia	[mækrəʊˈɡlɒsɪə] 巨舌
malocclusion	[ˌmæləˈkluːʒn] （牙）咬合不正
megacolon	[meɡəˈkəʊlən] 巨结肠（症）
nausea	[ˈnɔːzɪə] 恶心；反胃
proctocele	[pˈrɒktəʊseliː] 直肠膨出，直肠突出
proctoptosis	[prɒktɒpˈtəʊsɪs] 直肠脱垂
regurgitation	[rɪˌɡɜːdʒɪˈteɪʃn] 流回；逆流；反刍
splenomegaly	[ˌspliːnəʊˈmeɡəlɪ] 脾（肿）大
ulcer	[ˈʌlsə(r)] 溃疡
volvulus	[ˈvɒlvjʊləs] 肠扭转；肠扭结
vomiting	[ˈvɒmɪtɪŋ] 呕吐的
Zollinger-Ellision syndrome	佐林格-埃利森综合征

（三）消化系统检查术语

1. 消化系统内镜和非手术术语

表1-2-32 消化系统内镜和非手术表达术语表

消化系统内镜和非手术术语	中文释义
barium enema	钡灌肠
barium swallow	钡餐
cholangiography	[kəʊlændʒɪˈɒɡrəfɪ] 胆管造影术
cholecystography	[ˌkɒlɪsɪsˈtɒɡrəfɪ] 胆囊造影术
colonoscopy	[ˌkəʊləˈnɒskɒpɪ] 结肠镜检查
esophagoscopy	[iːsɒfəˈɡɒskəpɪ] 食管镜测法
esophagram	[iːˈsɒfəɡræm] 食管X线片
gastroscopy	[ɡæsˈtrɒskəpɪ] 胃镜检查法
laparoscopy	[ˌlæpəˈrɒskəpɪ] 腹腔镜检查
percutaneous transhepatic cholangiography	经皮肝穿胆管造影术

2. 消化系统手术术语

表 1-2-33 消化系统手术表达术语表

消化系统手术术语	中文释义
abdominocentesis	[æbˌdɒmɪnəsenˈtiːsɪs] 腹腔穿刺术
anoplasty	[ænɒpˈlæstɪ] 肛门成形术，肛修复术
appendectomy	[ˌæpenˈdektəmɪ] 阑尾切除术
cecocolostomy	[sɪkəʊkəˈlɒstəmɪ] 盲肠结肠吻合术
cecoileostomy	[sɪkɒɪˈliːəʊstəmɪ] 盲肠回肠吻合术
celioenterotomy	[siːliːəˈʊentərɒtəmɪ] 剖腹肠切开术
celiogastrotomy	[siːlaɪəʊgæstˈrəʊtəmɪ] 剖腹胃切开术
celiorrhaphy	[ˈsiːlɪərəfɪ] 腹壁缝术
celiotomy	[siːlɪˈɒtəmɪ] 剖腹手术；开腹术
cheiloplasty	[ˈkaɪləplæstɪ] 唇成形术
cheilorrhaphy	[kiːˈɒrəfɪ] 唇缝术，唇缝合术
cheilotomy	[kaɪˈlɒtəmɪ] 唇切开术
cholangioenterostomy	[kəʊlədʒiːəʊentəˈrɒstəmɪ] 胆管小肠吻合术，肝外胆道肠道吻合术
cholangiogastrostomy	[kəʊlæŋgiːəʊgæstˈrɒstəmɪ] 胆管胃吻合术
cholecystectomy	[ˌkɒlɪsɪsˈtektəmɪ] 胆囊切除术
cholecystolithotripsy	[ˈkəʊlsɪstəʊlɪθəʊtrɪps] 胆囊碎石术
cholecystopexy	[kəʊlsɪstəʊˈpeksɪ] 胆囊固定术
cholecystomy	[ˈkəʊlsɪstəmɪ] 胆囊切开术
choledocholithotomy	[ˈkəʊldɒkəlɪθəʊtəmɪ] 胆总管石切除术
cholelithotomy	[ˈˈkɒlɪlɪθəʊtəmɪ] 胆石切除术
colectomy	[kəˈlektəmɪ] 结肠切除术
colocentesis	[kəʊləsenˈtiːsɪs] 结肠穿刺术
colocolostomy	[kəʊləʊkəˈlɒstəmɪ] 肠结肠吻合术
colopexy	[kɒlɒˈpeksɪ] 结肠固定术
coloproctectomy	[kɒlɒprɒkˈtektəmɪ] 结肠直肠切除术
colostomy	[kəˈlɒstəmɪ] 结肠造口术
duodenectomy	[djuːəʊdɪˈnektəmɪ] 十二指肠切除术
duodenoenterostomy	[djuːədɪnəʊntəˈrɒstəmɪ] 十二指肠小肠造口吻合术

续表

消化系统手术术语	中文释义
duodenoileostomy	[djuədɪnɒɪˈliːəʊstəmɪ] 十二指肠回肠造口吻合术
duodenojejunostomy	[djuədɪnəʊdʒɪdʒuːˈnɒstəmɪ] 十二指肠空肠造口吻合术
duodenostomy	[djuədɪˈnɒstəmɪ] 十二指肠造口术
enteroanastomosis	[entərəʊənæstəˈməʊsɪs] 肠吻合术
enteropexy	[entərəʊˈpeksɪ] 肠固定术
enterostomy	[ˌentəˈrɒstəmɪ] 肠造口术
enterotomy	[ˌentəˈrɒtəmɪ] 肠切开术
esophagostomy	[iːsɒˈfeɪgəstəmɪ] 食管造口术
esophagotomy	[ɪsɒfəˈgɒtəmɪ] 食管切开术
gastrectomy	[gæsˈtrektəmɪ] 胃切除术
gastrocolostomy	[gæstrəʊkəˈlɒstəmɪ] 胃结肠吻合术
gastropexy	[gæstˈrəʊpeksɪ] 胃固定术
gastrorrhaphy	[gæstˈrɒrəfɪ] 胃缝术,胃修补术
gastrotomy	[gæsˈtrɒtəmɪ] 胃切开术
glossectomy	[glɒˈsektəmɪ] 舌截除术
glossorrhaphy	[glɒˈsɒrəfɪ] 舌缝术
hemorrhoidectomy	[ˌhemərɒɪˈdektəmɪ] 痔切除术
hepatectomy	[ˌhepəˈtektəmɪ] 肝切除术
hepatopexy	[ˈhepətəpeksɪ] 肝固定术
hepatorrhaphy	[hɪpeɪˈtɒrəfɪ] 肝缝术,肝缝合术
hernioplasty	[ˈhɜːnɪəplæstɪ] 疝根治手术
ileostomy	[ɪlɪˈɒstəmɪ] 回肠造口术
jejunostomy	[dʒɪdʒuːˈnɒstəmɪ] 空肠造口术
mesenteriopexy	[mesenˈterɪəpeksɪ] 肠系膜固定术
palatoplasty	[pæˈlɑːtɒplæstɪ] 腭成形术
pancreatectomy	[pæŋkrɪəˈtektəmɪ] 胰切除术
parotidectomy	[pərɒtɪˈdektəmɪ] 腮腺切除术
peritoneocentesis	[ˈperɪtəʊniːəʊsntɪzɪs] 腹腔穿刺
pharyngotomy	[ˌfærɪŋˈgɒtəmɪ] 咽切开(术)
proctectomy	[prɒkˈtektəmɪ] 直肠切除术

续表

消化系统手术术语	中文释义
proctopexy	[prɒktɒˈpeksɪ] 直肠固定术
proctostomy	[prɒkˈtəʊstəmɪ] 直肠造口术
proctotomy	[prɒkˈtɒtəmɪ] 直肠切开术
sialoadenotomy	[sˈləʊdenəʊtəmɪ] 涎腺切开术,涎腺切开引流术
sigmoidectomy	[sɪgmɒɪˈdektəmɪ] 乙状结肠切除术
sphinterotomy	[sfɪŋktəˈrɒtəmɪ] 括约肌切开术
stomatoplasty	[stəˈmætəplæstɪ] 口成形术,口腔成形术

3. 消化系统检查术语

表1-2-34 消化系统检查表达术语表

消化系统检查方式术语	中文释义
amylase	[ˈæmɪleɪz] 淀粉酶
fasting blood sugar（FBS）	空腹血糖
glucose tolerance test（GTS）	葡萄糖耐量试验
insulin clearance	胰岛素清除率
occult blood	潜血
serum bilirubin	血清胆红素
stool culture	便培养

（四）消化系统药学术语

表1-2-35 消化系统药学表达术语表

消化系统药学术语	意义
antacid	[æntˈæsɪd] 解酸剂
antidiarrheal	[ˈæntɪdəriːl] 止泻药
antiemetic	[æntɪmetɪk] 止吐剂
antinauseant	[ɒntɪˈnɔːsiːənt] 止恶心剂
antihistamine	[ˌæntɪˈhɪstəmiːn] 抗组胺剂
antispasmodic	[æntɪspæzˈmɒdɪk] 止痉挛药
cathartic	[kəˈθɑːtɪk] 泻药
emetic	[ɪˈmetɪk] 催吐剂

七、泌尿生殖系统

（一）泌尿生殖系统词根和组合形式

表 1-2-36 泌尿生殖系统词根和组合形式

泌尿生殖词根和组合形式	举例
balan/o-（the glans penis or the glans clitorids）	*balano*plasty [bælənɒpˈlæstɪ] 龟头成形术
crypt/o-（hidden, concealed）	*crypt*orchidism [krɪpˈtɔːkɪdɪzəm] 隐睾病
cyst/o-（sac, cyst, or bladder）	*cysto*cele [ˈsɪstəsiːl] 膀胱突出症
epididym/o-（epididymis）	*epididym*otomy [epɪdɪdɪˈmɒtmɪ] 附睾切开术
episi/o-（vulva）	*episio*stenosis [ɪpɪziːəʊsteˈnəʊsɪs] 外阴狭窄
gamet/o-（gamete）	*gameto*cyte [gəˈmiːtəsaɪt] 配子（母）细胞
gen/o-（reproduction, sex）	*geno*blast [ˈdʒenəblæst] 成熟性细胞
genit/o-（organs of reproduction）	*genito*plasty [dˈʒenɪtəplæstɪ] 生殖器成形术
glomerul/o-（glomerulus）	*glomerul*itis [glɒmerjʊˈlaɪtɪs] 肾小球炎
gon/o-（seed, semen）	*gono*cyte [ˈgɒnəsaɪt] 生殖母细胞
gonad/o-（gonad, ovary or testis）	*gonad*ectomy [gɒnæˈdektəmɪ] 性腺切除术
gravid/o-（pregnancy）	*gravido*cardiac [grəvɪdəʊˈkɑːdɪæk] 妊娠心脏病的
gyne-, gynaec/o-, gynec/o-, gyn/o- （woman or female sex） hysterodynia	*gyne*cology [ˌgaɪnɪˈkɒlədʒɪ] 妇科
hyster/o-（uterus）	*hystero*dynia [hɪstərəʊˈdɪnɪə] 子宫痛
men/o-（the menses）	*meno*pause [ˈmenəpɔːz] 停经期
metro-, mentra-（uterus）	*metro*endometritis [metrəʊndəʊˈmɪtraɪtɪs] 子宫体内膜炎
noct-（night）	*noct*uria [nɒkˈtjʊərɪə] 夜尿症；遗尿症
olig/o-（little）	*olig*uria [ɒlɪˈgjʊərɪə] 尿过少；少尿（症）
omphal/o-（navel）	*omphalo*cele [ˈɒmfələʊsiːl] 脐突出
oo-（egg）	*oo*blast [ˈəʊəblɑːst] 成卵细胞
oophor/o-（ovary）	*oophor*itis [ˌəʊəfəˈraɪtɪs] 卵巢炎
orchi/o-（testis）	*orchi*dectomy [ɔːkɪˈdektəmɪ] 睾丸切除术
ovari/o-（ovary）	*ovario*rrhexis [əʊveərɪəˈreksɪs] 卵巢破裂
papill/i-（papilla）	*papill*oma [ˌpæpɪˈləʊmə] 乳头状瘤；刺瘤

续表

泌尿生殖词根和组合形式	举例
phall/o-（penis）	*phall*ocrypsis [fæləʊkˈrɪpsɪs] 阴茎退缩
prostat/o-（prostate）	*prostat*omegaly [prɒsteɪˈtəmegəlɪ] 前列腺肥大
py/o-（pus）	*py*ometritis [paɪəmetˈraɪtɪs] 脓性子宫炎
pyel/o-（pelvis of kidney）	*pyel*onephritis [paɪələʊnɪˈfraɪtɪs] 肾盂肾炎
scrot/o-（scrotum）	*scrot*itis [ˈskrəʊˈtaɪtɪs] 阴囊炎
spermat/o-（sperm）	*spermat*olysis [ˌspɜːməˈtɒlɪsɪs] 精子溶解
test/o-（testis）	*test*itis [tesˈtaɪtɪs] 睾丸炎
toc/o-（childbirth or labor）	*toc*ophobia [təʊkəʊˈfəʊbɪə] 儿童恐怖
ureter/o-（ureter）	*ureter*ostenosis [jʊəriːtərʊsteˈnəʊsɪs] 输尿管狭窄
urethr/o-（urethra）	*urethr*ocystitis [jʊərəθrəsɪsˈtaɪtɪs] 尿道膀胱炎
vagin/o-（vagina）	*vagin*ocele [vædʒɪˈnəʊseliː] 阴道脱垂
vesic/o-（bladder）	*vesic*otomy [ˌvesɪˈkɒtəmɪ] 膀胱切开术
vulv/o-（vulva）	*vulv*itis [vʌlˈvaɪtɪs] 外阴炎

（二）泌尿生殖系统临床和病理术语

1. 泌尿生殖系统炎性和感染术语

表 1-2-37　泌尿生殖系统临床和病理表达术语表

泌尿生殖系统炎性和感染术语	中文释义
balanitis	[bæləˈnaɪtɪs] 龟头炎
bartholinitis	[bɑːθəʊlɪˈnɪtəs] 前庭大腺炎
cellulitis	[ˌseljʊˈlaɪtɪs] 蜂窝织炎
cervicitis	[ˌsɜːvɪˈsaɪtɪs] 子宫颈炎
chronic cystic mastitis	慢性囊性乳腺炎
cystitis	[sɪˈstaɪtɪs] 膀胱炎
endometritis	[ˌendəʊmɪˈtraɪtɪs] 子宫内膜炎
epididymitis	[ˌepɪˌdɪdɪˈmaɪtɪs] 附睾炎
glomerulonephritis	[glɒmerjʊləʊnefˈraɪtɪs] 肾小球性肾炎
mammillitis	[mæmɪˈlaɪtɪs] 乳头炎
mastadenitis	[mæstɑːˈdenaɪtɪs] 乳腺炎
metritis	[mɪˈtraɪtɪs] 子宫炎

续表

泌尿生殖系统炎性和感染术语	中文释义
metrophlebitis	[metrəʊflɪˈbaɪtɪs] 子宫静脉炎
metrosalpingitis	[metrəʊzɔːlpɪndˈʒaɪtɪs] 子宫输卵管炎
myometritis	[maɪəmetˈraɪtɪs] 子宫肌炎，子宫肌层炎
nephritis	[neˈfraɪtɪs] 肾炎
nephrotuberculosis	[nefrətəbɜːkjʊˈləʊsɪs] 肾结核
oophoritis	[ˌəʊəfəˈraɪtɪs] 卵巢炎
oophorosalpingitis	[uːfɒrəʊzælpɪndˈʒaɪtɪs] 卵巢输卵管炎
orchitis	[ɔːˈkaɪtɪs] 睾丸炎
parametritis	[pærəmɪˈtraɪtɪs] 子宫旁（组织）炎
perinephritis	[perɪnəˈfraɪtɪs] 肾周炎
perioophoritis	[perɪəʊfəˈraɪtɪs] 卵巢周炎
prostatitis	[ˌprɒstəˈtaɪtɪs] 前列腺炎
pyelitis	[ˌpaɪəˈlaɪtɪs] 肾盂炎
pyelocystitis	[paɪləsɪsˈtaɪtɪs] 膀胱肾盂炎，肾盂膀胱炎
pyelonephritis	[paɪələʊnɪˈfraɪtɪs] 肾盂肾炎
pyocolpos	[paɪəʊˈkɒlpəs] 阴道积脓
pyometra	[paɪəʊˈmiːtrə] 子宫积脓
pyonephritis	[paɪəʊnɪˈfraɪtɪs] 脓性肾炎
pyonephrosis	[paɪənɪˈfrəʊsɪs] 脓性肾病
pyosalpinx	[paɪəʊˈsælpɪŋks] 输卵管积脓
salpingitis	[ˌsælpɪnˈdʒaɪtɪs] 输卵管炎
ureteritis	[jʊəretəˈraɪtɪs] 输尿管炎
ureteropyosis	[jʊəriːtərəpaˈɪəʊsɪs] 输尿管化脓
urethritis	[ˌjʊərəˈθraɪtɪs] 尿道炎
urethrocystitis	[jʊəreθrəsɪsˈtaɪtɪs] 尿道膀胱炎
vaginitis	[ˌvædʒəˈnaɪtɪs] 阴道炎
vesiculitis	[vɪsɪkjʊˈlaɪtɪs] 精囊炎
vulvitis	[vʌlˈvaɪtɪs] 外阴炎

2. 泌尿生殖系统性病术语

表 1-2-38 泌尿生殖系统性病表达术语表

泌尿生殖系统性病术语	中文释义
acquired immune deficiency syndrome（AIDS）	艾滋病；获得性免疫功能丧失综合征
genital wart	湿疣
candidiasis	[ˌkændəˈdaɪəsəs] 念珠菌病
gonorrhea	[ˌɡɒnəˈriːə] 淋病
genital Herpes	生殖器疱疹
syphilis	[ˈsɪfɪlɪs] 梅毒
trichomoniasis	[ˌtrɪkəməˈnaɪəsɪs] 毛滴虫病

3. 泌尿生殖系统病理术语

表 1-2-39 泌尿生殖系统病理表达术语表

泌尿生殖系统病理术语	中文释义
abruptio placenta	胎盘早期脱离
albuminuria	[ælbjʊmɪnˈjuərɪə] 蛋白尿
amenorrhea	[eɪˌmenəˈriːə] 无月经；经闭
anarchism	[ˈænəkɪzəm] 无精症
anuria	[ənˈjuərɪə] 无尿，无尿症
aspermatogenesis	[æspəˈmətədʒiːnəsɪs] 精子生成缺乏症
aspermia	[ˈæspəmɪə] 无精，精液缺乏
aresia of vagina	阴道闭锁
azotemia	[æzəˈtiːmɪə] 氮血；氮血症；氮质血症
carcinoma of cervix	宫颈癌
cryptorchism	[krɪpˈtɔːkɪzəm] 隐睾病
cylindruria	[sɪlɪnˈdrʊərɪə] 管型尿
cystocele	[ˈsɪstəsiːl] 膀胱突出症
Displacement of uterus retroflexion, retroversion, or anteflexion	子宫前屈、后屈或前屈移位
dysmenorrhea	[ˌdɪsmenəʊˈriːə] 痛经
dyspareunia	[dɪspəˈruːnɪə] 性交困难
dysuria	[dɪsˈjʊərɪə] 排尿困难

续表

泌尿生殖系统病理术语	中文释义
epispadias	[epɪˈspeɪdɪəs] 尿道上裂
gynecomastia	[gaɪnɪkəʊˈmæstɪə] 男子女性型乳房
hematocolpos	[hiːmətəʊˈkɒlpɒs] 阴道积血
hematometra	[heməˈtəmetrə] 子宫积血,子宫经血滞留
hematosalpinx	[heməˈtəʊzælpɪŋks] 输卵管积血
hematuria	[ˌhiːməˈtjuːrɪə] 血尿症；血尿
hermaphroditism	[hɜːˈmæfrədaɪtɪzəm] 雌雄同体性
Hydatidiform mole	葡萄胎,水泡状胎块
hydronephrosis	[ˌhaɪdrənɪˈfrəʊsɪs] 肾盂积水
hypercalciuria	[haɪpəˈkælsɪərɪə] 尿钙过多,尿钙增多症,高钙尿
Hyperplasia of the endometrium	子宫内膜增
hypospadias	[haɪpəˈspeɪdɪəs] 尿道下裂
hysterolith	[ˈhɪstərəlɪθ] 子宫石
hysterorrhexis	[hɪstərəʊˈreksɪs] 子宫破裂
impotence	[ˈɪmpətəns] 阳痿
incontinence	[ɪnˈkɒntɪnəns] 失禁
leukorrhea	[ˌluːkəˈriːə] 白带
mastalgia	[mæsˈtældʒɪə] 乳腺痛
mastoptosis	[mɑːsˈtɒptəʊsɪs] 乳房下垂
mastorrhagia	[mæstəʊˈreɪdʒɪə] 乳腺出血
menometrorrhagia	[menəmetrəˈreɪdʒɪə] 月经过多
menoschesis	[məˈnɒskɪsɪs] 经闭；月经潴留
metratrophia	[metˈrætrɒfaɪə] 子宫萎缩
metrorrhagia	[ˌmiːtrəˈreɪdʒɪə] 子宫出血
metrostenosis	[metrɒsteˈnəʊsɪs] 子宫狭窄
nephrolith	[ˈnefrəlɪθ] 肾结石
nephrolithiasis	[nefrəʊlɪˈθaɪəsɪs] 肾石病
nephromegaly	[nefrəʊˈmegəlɪ] 巨肾
nephroptosis	[nefrɒpˈtəʊsɪs] 肾下垂
nephrosclerosis	[nefrəsklɪəˈrəʊsɪs] 肾硬化；肾硬变(症)

续表

泌尿生殖系统病理术语	中文释义
nephrosis	[nɪˈfrəʊsɪs] 肾变病；肾病
nephrorrhagia	[nefrɒˈrædʒə] 肾出血
oligohydramnios	[ɒlɪgəʊhaɪdˈræmniːəʊz] 羊水过少
oligomenorrhea	[ɒlɪgɒmɪnɒːˈrɪə] 经量减少，月经过少
oligospermia	[ɒlaɪˈgɒspəmɪə] 精子减少，精液缺乏
oliguria	[ɒlɪˈgjʊərɪə] 尿过少；少尿（症）
ovotestis	[ˌəʊvəˈtestɪs] 卵精巢；卵睾
phimosis	[faɪˈməʊsɪs] 包茎；包皮过长
phosphaturia	[fɒsfəˈtjʊərɪə] 高磷酸盐尿
polymastia	[ˌpɒlɪˈmæstɪə] 多乳房畸形
polyorchism	[pəʊlˈjɔːkɪzəm] 多睾
polythelia	[ˌpɒlɪˈθiːljə] 多乳头
polyuria	[ˌpɒlɪˈjʊərɪə] 多尿（症）
premenstrual syndrome（**PMS**）	经前综合征
prolapse of the uterus	子宫脱垂
prostatic hypertrophy	前列腺肥大症
pseudohermaphroditism	[sjuːdəʊhəˈmæfrədɪtɪs] 假两性畸形，假雌雄同体现象
puerperal eclampsia	子痫
pyelonephrosis	[paɪləʊˈnefrəʊsɪs] 肾盂肾病
pyuria	[paɪˈjʊərɪə] 脓尿
seminoma	[semɪˈnəʊmə] 精原细胞瘤
spermatocele	[ˈspɜːmətəʊsiːl] 精液囊肿
spermaturia	[ˌspɜːməˈtjʊərɪə] 精液尿
spontaneous abortion	自发性流产
sterility	[stəˈrɪlətɪ] 不生育
synorchidism	[sɪˈnɔːkɪdɪzəm] 睾丸粘连
teratoma	[ˌterəˈtəʊmə] 畸胎瘤
thecoma	[θɪˈkəʊmə] 泡膜细胞瘤
uraturia	[jʊəˈreɪtərɪə] 尿酸尿
uremia	[jʊˈriːmɪə] 尿毒症

续表

泌尿生殖系统病理术语	中文释义
ureteralgia	[juəriˈtəˈrældʒə] 输尿管痛
ureterectasis	[juəjuə:tɪˈrektəsɪs] 输尿管扩张
ureterolith	[ˈjuəri:tərəlɪθ] 输尿管石
ureterolithiasis	[juəri:tərəlɪˈθaɪəsɪs] 输尿管石病
ureterolysis	[juəri:təˈrɒlɪsɪs] 输尿管松解术
ureterorrhagia	[juəri:tˈrɒrædʒə] 输尿管出血
ureterostenosis	[juəri:tərɒsteˈnəusɪs] 输尿管狭窄
urethralgia	[juəri:θˈrældʒə] 尿道痛
urethremphraxis	[juəjuəθˈremfræksɪs] 尿道梗阻
urethrorrhagia	[juəreθˈrɒrædʒə] 尿道出血
urethrorrhea	[juəˈreθrɒrɪə] 尿道液溢
urethrostaxis	[juəreθrəʊsˈtæksɪs] 尿道渗血
vaginismus	[ˌvædʒɪˈnɪzməs] 阴道痉挛
varicocele	[ˈværɪkəʊsi:l] 静脉节瘤

（三）泌尿生殖系统检查术语

表 1-2-40　泌尿生殖系统检查表达术语表

泌尿生殖系统检查术语	中文释义
addis count	艾迪斯计数
amniocentesis	[ˌæmnɪəʊsenˈti:sɪs] 羊膜穿刺术
amniography	[æmniˈɔʊɡrəfɪ] 羊膜造影术
chorionic vil li sampling（*CVS*）	绒毛标本采取
creatinine test	肌酐测试
cystogram	[ˈsɪstəɡræm] 膀胱造影片
endogenous creatinine clearance rate	内生肌酸酐清除率
hemoglobin test	血红蛋白测试
hysterogram	[ˈhɪstərəɡræm] 子宫造影片
hysteroscopy	[hɪstəˈrɒskəpɪ] 子宫镜检查（术）
intravenous pyelogram	静脉肾盂造影
karyotyping	[ˈkærɪəˌtaɪp] 染色体组型
mammography	[mæˈmɒɡrəfɪ] 乳房 X 线照相术

续表

泌尿生殖系统检查术语	中文释义
radioreceptor assay	放射性受体测定
renal scan	肾扫描
retrograde pyelogram	逆行性肾盂造影片
seminal fluid tests	精液测试
urine total volume	总尿量

（四）泌尿生殖系统手术术语

表1-2-41　泌尿生殖系统手术表达术语表

泌尿生殖系统手术术语	中文释义
abortion	[əˈbɔːʃn] 流产；堕胎
amniotomy	[æmnaˈɪəutəumɪ] 羊膜穿破术
cervicectomy	[sɜːvɪˈsektəmɪ] 子宫颈切除术
cesarean section	剖宫产术
circumcision	[ˌsɜːkəmˈsɪʒn] 包皮环切（术）
clitoridectomy	[klɪtɔːraɪˈdektəmɪ] 阴蒂切除术
colpectomy	[kɒlˈpektəmɪ] 阴道切除术
colpocleisis	[kɒlpəʊkˈlɪaɪzɪs] 阴道闭合术
colpomyomectomy	[kɒlpəmaɪəˈmektəmɪ] 阴道式子宫肌瘤切除术
colpoperineoplasty	[kɒlpəʊpərɪniːəʊˈlæstaɪ] 阴道会阴成形术
colpoperineorrhaphy	[kɒlpəʊpərɪˈnɔːrəfɪ] 阴道会阴缝术
colpopexy	[kɒlpəʊˈpeksɪ] 阴道固定术
colpoplasty	[kɒlˈpəʊplæstaɪ] 阴道成形术
colpopoiesis	[ˈkɒlpəpɒiːsɪs] 阴道造形术
cystidolaparotomy	[sɪstaɪdəʊləpæˈrəʊtəmɪ] 剖腹膀胱切开术
cystidotrachelotomy	[sɪstɪdətræʃˈləʊtəumɪ] 膀胱颈切开术
cystolithectomy	[sɪstəʊlɪˈθektəmɪ] 膀胱石切除术
cystopexy	[sɪstəʊˈpeksɪ] 膀胱固定术
cystoplasty	[sɪstəpˈlæstɪ] 膀胱成形术
cystoproctostomy	[sɪstɒprɒkˈtəʊstəmɪ] 膀胱直肠造口吻合术
cystorrhaphy	[sɪsˈtɔːrəfɪ] 膀胱缝合术

续表

泌尿生殖系统手术术语	中文释义
cystostomy	[sɪsˈtɒstəmɪ] 膀胱造口术
cystotomy	[sɪsˈtɒtəmɪ] 膀胱切开术
dilatation and curettage (*D&C*)	宫颈扩张子宫刮术
epididymectomy	[epɪdaɪdɪˈmektəmɪ] 附睾切除术
epididymotomy	[epɪdɪdɪˈmɒtəmɪ] 附睾切开术
epididymovasostomy	[epɪdaɪdɪmuːˈveɪsɒstəmɪ] 输精管附睾吻合术
episioplasty	[ɪpɪzaɪɒpˈlæstɪ] 外阴成形术
episiorrhaphy	[ˈɪpɪzɪərəfɪ] 外阴缝合术
episiotomy	[ɪˌpiːsɪˈɒtəmɪ] 外阴切开术
hemodialysis	[ˌhiːmədaɪˈælɪsɪs] 血液透析
hymenectomy	[hɪmˈnektəmɪ] 处女膜切除术
hysterectomy	[ˌhɪstəˈrektəmɪ] 子宫切除（术)
hysteromyotomy	[hɪstərəˈmaɪəʊtəmɪ] 子宫肌切开术
hysteropexy	[hɪstəˈrɒpeksɪ] 子宫固定术
hysterorrhaphy	[hɪstəˈrɒrəfɪ] 子宫缝合术
hysterosalpingostomy	[hɪstərəsælpɪŋˈgɒstəmɪ] 子宫输卵管吻合术
mastectomy	[mæˈstektəmɪ] 乳房切除术
mastopexy	[ˈmæstəpeksɪ] 乳房固定术
mastoplasty	[ˈmæstəplæstɪ] 乳房成形术
mastotomy	[mæsˈtɒtəmɪ] 乳房切开术
nephrocystanastomosis	[nefrəsɪstənəstəˈməʊzɪ] 肾膀胱吻合术
nephrolithotomy	[nefrəʊlɪˈθɒtəmɪ] 肾石切开术
nephrostomy	[nɪˈfrɒstəmɪ] 肾造口术
nephrotomy	[neˈfrɒtəmɪ] 肾切开术
nephroureterectomy	[nefrəretɪˈrektəmɪ] 肾输尿管切除术
nephroureterocystectomy	[nefrəretərəsɪsˈtekt] 肾输尿管膀胱切除术
oophorectomy	[ˌəʊəfəˈrektəmɪ] 卵巢切除术
oophorocystectomy	[uːfɒrəsɪsˈtektəmɪ] 卵巢囊肿切除术
oophorohysterectomy	[uːfɒrəʊhɪstɪˈrektəmɪ] 卵巢子宫切除术
oophoropexy	[uːfɒrəʊˈpeksɪ] 卵巢固定术

续表

泌尿生殖系统手术术语	中文释义
oophoroplasty	[uːˈfɒrəʊplæstaɪ] 卵巢成形术
oophorosalpingectomy	[uːfɒrəʊzælpɪndˈʒektəmɪ] 卵巢输卵管切除术
oophorotomy	[uːfɒˈrəʊtəmɪ] 卵巢切开术
orchidopexy	[ˈɔːkɪdəʊpeksɪ] 睾丸固定术
orchiectomy	[ɔːkɪˈektəmɪ] 睾丸切除术
orchioplasty	[ɔːtʃaɪɒpˈlæstɪ] 睾丸成形术
ovariocentesis	[əʊˌvɑːriːəʊsentɪzɪs] 卵巢穿刺术
ovariostomy	[əʊˈvɑːriːəʊstəmɪ] 卵巢造口术
ovariotomy	[əʊveərɪˈɒtəmɪ] 卵巢切开术
prostatectomy	[prɒstəˈtektəmɪ] 前列腺切除术
prostatomy	[prɒsˈteɪtəmɪ] 前列腺切开术
prostatovesiculectomy	[prɒstətəʊvesɪkjuːˈlektɒm] 前列腺精囊切除术
pyelolithotomy	[paɪələʊlɪˈθɒtəmɪ] 肾盂石切除术
pyeloplasty	[paɪləʊpˈlæstɪ] 肾盂成形术
salpingectomy	[ˌsælpɪnˈdʒektəmɪ] 输卵管切除术
salpingopexy	[sælpɪnˈgəʊpeksɪ] 输卵管固定术
salpingostomatomy	[sælpɪngəstəmˈtəmɪ] 输卵管部分切除造口术
salpingotomy	[sælpɪnˈgɒtəmɪ] 输卵管切除术
scrotoplasty	[skˈrəʊtəplæstɪ] 阴囊成形术
trachelorrhaphy	[trækəˈlɔːrəfɪ] 子宫颈缝合术
trachelotomy	[trəʃˈeləʊtəʊmɪ] 子宫颈切开术
ureterectomy	[jʊəriːtəˈrektəmɪ] 输尿管切除术
ureterocystanastomosis	[jʊəriːtərəsɪsˈtənəstəməʊz] 输尿管膀胱吻合术
ureterolithotomy	[jʊəriːtərəʊlɪˈθɒtəmɪ] 输尿管石切除术
ureteroneopyelostomy	[jʊəriːtəwʌˈniːpaɪləstəmɪ] 输尿管肾盂吻合术
ureteroplasty	[jʊəriːtərəpˈlæstɪ] 输尿管成形术
ureterorrhaphy	[jʊəriːtˈrɒrəfɪ] 输尿管缝合术
ureterostomy	[jʊˌriːtəˈrəʊstəmɪ] 输尿管造口术
ureteroureterostomy	[jʊəriːtəretəˈrɒstəmɪ] 输尿管吻合术
ureteroproctostomy	[jʊəriːtərəprɒkˈtəʊstəmɪ] 输尿管直肠吻合术

续表

泌尿生殖系统手术术语	中文释义
urethrocystopexy	[juərəθrəsɪstəʊˈpeksɪ] 尿道膀胱固定术
urethroplasty	[jʊəˈriːθrəplæstɪ] 尿道成形术
urethrorrhaphy	[juərəθˈrɒrəfɪ] 尿道缝合术
urethrostomy	[juərəθˈrɒstəmɪ] 尿道造口术
urethrotomy	[ˌjʊərəˈθrɒtəmɪ] 尿道切开术
vasectomy	[vəˈsektəmɪ] 输精管切除
vesiculectomy	[vəsɪkjuːˈlektəmɪ] 囊切除术
vesiculotomy	[vəsɪkjʊˈləʊtəmɪ] 精囊切开术
vulvectomy	[vʌlˈvektəmɪ] 外阴切除术

（五）泌尿生殖系统药学术语

表 1-2-42　泌尿生殖系统药学表达术语表

泌尿生殖系统药学术语	中文释义
contraceptive	[ˌkɒntrəˈseptɪv] 避孕药
oxytocin	[ˌɒksɪˈtəʊsɪn] 催产素
spermicide	[ˈspɜːmɪsaɪd] 杀精子剂

八、神经系统

（一）神经系统词根和组合形式

表 1-2-43　神经系统词根和组合形式表

神经系统词根/组合形式/后缀	举例
amnio-（amnion）	*amnio*scopy [ˈæmniːəʊskɒpɪ] 羊膜镜检查法
arachn/o-（arachnoid membrane）	*arachno*iditis [æræknɒɪˈdaɪtɪs] 蛛网膜眼
astr/o-, aster/o-（star-shaped）	*astro*cyte [ˈæstrəsaɪt] 星型细胞
cerebell/o-（cerebellum）	*cerebell*itis [seɪəbeˈlɪtɪs] 小脑炎
cry/o-（cold）	*cryo*surgery [ˌkraɪəʊˈsɜːdʒərɪ] 冷冻手术
encephala/o-（brain）	*encephal*opathy [enˌsefəˈlɒpəθɪ] 脑病
gangli/o-, ganglion/o-（ganglion）	*gangli*oma [gæŋglɪˈəʊmə] 神经节瘤
gli/o-（gluey substance）	*glio*cyte [ˈglaɪəʊsaɪt] 胶质细胞

续表

神经系统词根/组合形式/后缀	举例
kinesi/o-, *kine-*（movement）	*kinesi*therapy [kaɪniːsɪˈθerəpɪ] 运动疗法
medull/o-（medulla）	*medull*ectomy [medʌˈlektəmɪ] 髓质切除术
mening/o-（membrane）	*mening*ococcus [məˌnɪŋəˈkɒkəs] 脑膜炎球菌
myel/o-（marrow）	*myel*ocele [ˈmaɪələʊsiːl] 脊髓突出
myelin/o-（a white fatty material）	*myelin*opathy [ˈmaɪlɪnəpəθɪ] 髓鞘质病
narc/o-（numbness）	*narc*oma [nɑːˈkəʊmə] 昏睡
syring/o-（tube, fistula）	*syring*ocele [sɪˈrɪɡəʊsiːl] 空洞性脊髓突出
spin/o-（spine）	*spin*algia [spaɪˈnældʒɪə] 脊椎痛
-lepsy（seizure）	psycho*lepsy* [saɪˈkɒlepsɪ] 精神猝变
-lexia（speech）	a*lexia* [əˈleksɪə] 失读症
-taxia（muscular coordination）	a*taxia* [əˈtæksɪə] 运动失调

（二）神经系统临床和病理术语

表 1-2-44 神经系统炎症和感染表达术语表

神经系统炎症和感染术语	中文释义
arachnoiditis	[ærækno̞ɪˈdaɪtɪs] 蛛网膜炎
choriomeningitis	[kɔːrɪəʊmenɪnˈdʒaɪtɪs] 脉络丛脑膜炎
encephalitis	[enˌsefəˈlaɪtəs] 脑炎
encephalomyelitis	[enˌsefələʊmaɪəˈlaɪtɪs] 脑脊髓炎
ependymitis	[ependɪˈmaɪtɪs] 脑室管膜炎
ganglionitis	[ˈɡæŋɡlɪənaɪtɪs] 神经节炎
herpes zoster	[ˌhɜːpiːzˈzɒstə(r)] 带状疱疹
leptomeningitis	[leptəmenɪˈdʒaɪtɪs] 柔脑（脊）膜炎
meningitis	[ˌmenɪnˈdʒaɪtɪs] 脑（脊）膜炎
meningoencephalitis	[mɪˌnɪŋɡəʊnsefəˈlaɪtɪs] 脑膜脑炎
meningoencephalomyelitis	[ˈmenɪŋɡəʊnsefələmaɪəˈlaɪtɪs] 脑膜脑脊髓炎
meningomyelitis	[mɪnɪŋɡəʊmaɪəˈlaɪtɪs] 脊膜脊髓炎
myelitis	[ˌmaɪəˈlaɪtɪs] 脊髓炎
myelosyphilis	[maɪələˈsɪfɪlɪs] 脊髓梅毒
neuritis	[njʊəˈraɪtɪs] 神经炎

续表

神经系统炎症和感染术语	中文释义
neuromyelitis	[njuərəmaˈɪəlaɪtɪz] 神经脊髓炎
pachyleptomeningitis	[pækɪleptʊmenɪndˈʒaɪtɪs] 硬软脑[脊]膜炎
polioencephalomeningomyelitis	[ˈpəʊliːəʊənkefələʊmeaɪlaɪtɪs] 脑脊髓灰质脑脊膜炎
poliomyelitis	[ˌpəʊlɪəʊˌmaɪəˈlaɪtɪs] 脊髓灰质炎；小儿麻痹症
poliomyeloencephalitis	[pəʊliːəʊmaɪˈləʊnkefəlaɪtɪs] 脑脊髓灰质炎
polyneuritis	[ˌpɒlɪnjʊˈraɪtɪs] 多神经炎
rabies	[ˈreɪbiːz] 狂犬病
radiculitis	[rædɪkjʊˈlaɪtɪs] 脊神经根炎
Reye's Syndrome	Reye 综合征
Tetanus	[ˈtetənəs] 破伤风

（三）神经系统精神术语

表 1-2-45 神经系统精神表达术语表

神经系统精神术语	中文释义
alcoholism	[ˈælkəhɒlɪzəm] 酒精中毒
anorexia nervosa	神经性厌食症
bipolar disorder	躁郁症
borderline personality disorder	边缘型人格异常
depression	[dɪˈpreʃn] 抑郁
hysteria	[hɪˈstɪərɪə] 歇斯底里症
major depression disorder	Major depression disorder
mania	[ˈmeɪnɪə] 躁狂
neurosis	[njʊəˈrəʊsɪs] 神经症；神经衰弱症
obsessive compulsive disorder	强迫症
paranoia	[ˌpærəˈnɒɪə] 偏执狂；妄想狂
personality disorder	病态人格
phobia	[ˈfəʊbɪə] 恐怖症
psychosis	[saɪˈkəʊsɪs] 精神病
schizophrenia	[ˌskɪtsəˈfriːnɪə] 精神分裂症

(四)神经系统病理术语

表 1-2-46 神经系统病理表达术语表

神经系统病理术语	中文释义
alexia	[əˈleksɪə] 失读症
Alzheimer's disease	老年痴呆症
amentia	[əˈmenʃɪə] 智力缺陷
amnesia	[æmˈniːzɪə] 健忘症
analgesia	[ˌænəlˈdʒiːzɪə] 痛觉缺失
anencephaly	[ænənˈsefəlɪ] 无脑畸形
apathy	[ˈæpəθɪ] 冷漠
aphasia	[əˈfeɪzɪə] 失语症
asthenia	[æsˈθiːnɪə] 无力;虚弱
astrocytoma	[ˌæstrəʊsaɪˈtəʊmə] 星形细胞瘤
ataxia	[əˈtæksɪə] 运动失调
atelencephalia	[ətelenseˈfəlɪə] 脑发育不全
atelomyelia	[əteləmɪˈiːlɪə] 脊髓发育不全
athetosis	[əˈðetəʊsɪs] 指痉症,徐动症
autism	[ˈɔːtɪzəm] 自闭症;孤独症
cataphasia	[kætəˈfeɪzɪə] 言语重复(症)
cephalagia	[seˈfɑːlɪdʒə] 头疼,头痛
cerebral hemorrhage	脑出血
cerebral palsy	大脑性麻痹
cerebrovascular accident	脑血管意外
chorea	[kəˈrɪə] 舞蹈病
coma	[ˈkəʊmə] 昏迷
craniomeningocele	[kreɪnɪɒmenɪŋɡəʊseliː] 颅部脑膜膨出
delirium	[dɪˈlɪrɪəm] 精神错乱;说胡话;狂喜
delusion	[dɪˈluːʒn] 错觉;幻觉
dementia	[dɪˈmenʃə] 痴呆
diplegia	[daɪˈpliːdʒɪə] 双侧瘫痪
dipsomania	[ˌdɪpsəʊˈmeɪnɪə] 嗜酒狂
disorientation	[dɪsˌɔːrɪenˈteɪʃn] 迷失方向;定向障碍

续表

神经系统病理术语	中文释义
drug dependency	赖药性，药瘾
dysarthria	[dɪsˈɑːrɪə] 构音困难；构音障碍
dysbasia	[dɪsˈbeɪzjə] 步行困难
dyskinesia	[ˌdɪskɪˈniːʒə] 运动障碍
dyslexia	[dɪsˈleksɪə] 阅读障碍
dysphasia	[dɪsˈfeɪzɪə] 言语障碍症
dyspraxia	[dɪsˈpræksɪə] 运动困难
encephalomalacia	[enˌsefələuməˈleɪʃɪə] 脑软化
encephalomyelocele	[ˈenkefələmaɪləuseliː] 脑脊髓膨出
epidural hematoma	硬膜外血肿
epilepsy	[ˈepɪlepsɪ] 癫痫症
euphoria	[juːˈfɔːrɪə] 幸福愉快感
exhibitionism	[ˌeksɪˈbɪʃənɪzəm] 暴露癖
gangliocytoma	[gæŋglaɪɒsaɪˈtəmə] 神经节细胞瘤
ganglioglioma	[gæŋglˈɪɒlɪəmə] 神经节神经胶质瘤
glioma	[glaɪˈəumə] 神经胶质瘤
hallucination	[həˌluːsɪˈneɪʃn] 幻觉；幻想
hemiplegia	[ˌhemɪˈpliːdʒɪə] 偏瘫；半身不遂
homosexuality	[ˌhɒməˌsekʃuˈælətɪ] 同性恋
hydrencephalocele	[haɪdrensefəˈləusiːl] 积水性脑突出
hydrocephalus	[ˈhaɪdrəuˈsefələs] 脑水肿；脑积水
hydromeningocele	[haɪdrəmeˈnɪŋgəsiːl] 积水性脑膜突出
hydromyelocele	[haɪdrəˈmaɪələsiːl] 积水性脊髓膜突出
hypochondria	[ˌhaɪpəˈkɒndrɪə] 疑病症；忧郁症
intracranial hemorrhage	颅内出血
lethargy	[ˈleθədʒɪ] 昏睡
macrocephaly	[mækrəuˈsefəlɪ] 巨头；巨头畸形
masochism	[ˈmæsəkɪzəm] 受虐狂；受虐倾向；性受虐
meningocele	[məˈnɪŋgəsiːl] 脑（脊）膜突出
meningoencephalocele	[menɪnˈgəunkefələuseliː] 脑脑膜突出

第一部分 医学英语

续表

神经系统病理术语	中文释义
meningomyelocele	[ˈmenɪŋɡəʊmaɪləʊseliː] 脑脊膜脊髓膨出
microcephaly	[ˌmaɪkrəʊˈsefəlɪ] 头小畸形
myelocele	[ˈmaɪələʊsiːl] 脊髓突出
myelodysplasia	[maɪələʊdɪˈspleɪzɪə] 脊髓发育不良
myelopathy	[maɪəˈlɒpəθɪ] 脊髓病
myeloschisis	[maɪəˈlɒskɪsɪs] 脊髓裂
narcissism	[ˈnɑːsɪsɪzəm] 自我陶醉；自恋
necromania	[nekrəʊˈneɪnɪə] 恋尸狂；恋尸癖
neurocytoma	[njʊərəsaɪˈtəʊmə] 神经细胞瘤
neurofibroma	[ˌnjʊərəʊfaɪˈbrəʊmə] 纤维神经瘤
neurofibromatosis	[njuəˈrəʊfaɪbrəʊmətəʊsɪs] 神经纤维瘤病
neuroglioma	[ˌnjʊərəɡlaɪˈəʊmə] 神经胶质瘤
palmomental reflex	掌颏反射
paralysis	[pəˈræləsɪs] 瘫痪；麻痹
paraparesis	[ˌpærəpəˈriːsɪs] 下身轻瘫；下肢轻瘫
paraphasia	[ˌpærəˈfeɪzjə] 语言错乱，错语症
paraplegia	[ˌpærəˈpliːdʒə] 半身不遂
Parkinson's disease	帕金森病；震颤性麻痹
petit mal	癫痫小发作
pica	[ˈpaɪkə] 异食癖
porencephaly	[pərənkeˈfeɪlɪ] 孔洞脑畸形，脑穿通畸形
pragmatagnosia	[præɡmætæɡˈnəʊzɪə] 物体认识不能，物体失认
spina biffda	脊柱裂
spongioblastoma	[ˈspʌndʒɪəʊblæsˈtəʊmə] 成胶质细胞瘤
stress	[stres] 压力
subarachnoid hemorrhage	蛛网膜下出血
subdural hemorrhage	硬脑膜下出血
syncope	[ˈsɪŋkəpɪ] 昏厥
sucking reflex	吸吮反射
syringobulbia	[sɪrɪˈɡəʊbʌlbɪə] 延髓空洞症

续表

神经系统病理术语	中文释义
tic	[tɪk] 痉挛；抽筋
torpor	[ˈtɔːpə(r)] 麻木；无感觉
voyeurism	[vɒɪˈɜːrɪzəm] 窥阴癖者
xanthochromia	[zænθəʊkˈrəʊmɪə] 黄变症

（五）神经系统检查术语

表 1-2-47　神经系统检查表达术语表

神经系统检查术语	中文释义
cerebral angiography	脑血管造影术
cerebrospinal fluid test	脑脊液检测
cordectomy	[kɒˈdektəmɪ] 索带切除术
craniotomy	[ˌkreɪnɪˈɒtəmɪ] 颅骨切开术；穿颅术
cranioplasty	[kreɪniːəʊpˈlæstɪ] 头颅成形术
cryosurgery	[ˌkraɪəʊˈsɜːdʒərɪ] 冷冻手术
echoencephalogram	[eˈkəʊnkefəlɒgræm] 脑回波图
electroencephalography	[ɪˈlektrəʊensefəˈlɒgrəfɪ] 脑电图学
encephalopuncture	[enkefəˈləʊpʌŋktʃə] 脑穿刺术
gangliectomy	[gæŋˈliːktəmɪ] 神经节切除术
laminectomy	[ˌlæmɪˈnektəmɪ] 椎板切除术
leucotomy	[luːˈkɒtəmɪ] 前额脑白质切除手术
myelography	[maɪˈlɒgrəfɪ] 脊髓造影术
neurectomy	[njʊˈrektəmɪ] 神经切除术
neuroanastomosis	[njʊərəʊnæstəˈməʊsɪs] 神经吻合术
neurolysis	[njʊəˈrɒlɪsɪs] 神经组织崩溃
neuroplasty	[njʊəˈrɒplæstɪ] 神经成形术
neurorrhaphy	[njuːˈrɒrəfɪ] 神经缝术
neurotomy	[njʊəˈrɒtəmɪ] 神经切断术
pneumoencephalography	[njuːməensɪfəˈlɒgrəfɪ] 气脑造影术
rachicentesis	[ˈrəʃɪsəntɪzɪs] 腰椎穿刺
Serum ammonia	血氨

续表

神经系统检查术语	中文释义
sympathectomy	[ˌsɪmpəˈθektəmɪ] 交感神经切除术
tendon reflex	腱反射
thalamotomy	[θæləˈmɒtəmɪ] 丘脑切开术
vagotomy	[vəˈgɒtəmɪ] 迷走神经切断术

（六）神经系统药学术语

表1-2-48 神经系统药学表达术语表

神经系统药学术语	意义
adrenergic	[ˌædrəˈnɜːdʒɪk] 肾上腺素
analgesic	[ˌænəlˈdʒiːzɪk] 镇痛剂
antianxiety drugs	抗焦虑药
anticonvulsant	[ˌæntɪkənˈvʌlsənt] 抗痉挛药，镇痉剂
antidepressant	[ˌæntɪdɪˈpresnt] 抗抑郁剂
antimaniacal	[ænti:məˈnaɪəkəl] 抗躁狂剂
cholinergic	[ˌkəʊlɪˈnɜːdʒɪk] 类胆碱（功）能的
hypnotic	[hɪpˈnɒtɪk] 催眠药；安眠药
opiate	[ˈəʊpɪeɪt] 鸦片剂；麻醉剂
parasympatholytic	[pærəsɪmpəθəʊˈlɪtɪk] 副交感神经阻断药
sedative	[ˈsedətɪv] 镇静剂
sympatholytic	[ˌsɪmpəθəʊˈlɪtɪk] 抗交感神经药
tranquilizer	[ˈtræŋkwɪlaɪzə] 镇静剂

九、内分泌系统

（一）内分泌系统词根和组合形式

表1-2-49 内分泌系统词根和组合形式表

词根/组合形式/后缀	举例
andr/o-（man or male）	**andro**gen [ˈændrədʒən] 雄激素
adren/o-（adrenal gland）	**adreno**kinetic [ədrenəkaɪˈnetɪk] 激肾上腺的
gluc/o-（sweet, glucose）	**gluco**protein [ˌgluːkəʊˈprəʊtiːn] 糖蛋白

续表

词根/组合形式/后缀	举例
glyc/o-（sweet, glucose）	*glyco*suria [ˌglaɪkəʊˈsjʊərɪə] 糖尿；糖尿病
parathyroid/o-（parathyroid gland）	*parathyroid*ectomy [pærəθaɪrɒɪˈdektəmɪ] 甲状旁腺切除术
thym/o-（thymus）	*thymo*lysis [θaɪˈmɒlɪsɪs] 胸腺溶解
thy/o-, thye/o-（thyroid gland）	*thy*rocele [ˈθaɪrəsiːl] 甲状腺肿
thyroid/o-（thyroid gland）	*thyroid*ism [ˈθaɪrɒɪdɪzəm] 甲状腺剂中毒
-phylaxis（protection）	ana*phylaxis* [ˌænəfɪˈlæksɪs] 过敏性反应
-tropin（stimulation）	somato*tropin* [ˌsəʊmətəʊˈtrəʊpɪn] 生长激素
-trophy（nutrition）	hyper*trophy* [haɪˈpɜːtrəfɪ] 肥大

（二）内分泌系统临床和病理术语

1. 内分泌系统炎症和感染术语

表 1-2-50　内分泌系统炎症和感染术语表达术语表

内分泌系统炎症和感染术语	中文释义
adrenalitis	[ədreˈnælaɪtɪz] 肾上腺炎
thyroiditis	[ˌθaɪrɒɪˈdaɪtɪs] 甲状腺炎

2. 内分泌系统病理术语

表 1-2-51　内分泌系统病理表达术语表

内分泌系统病理术语	中文释义
Addison's disease	爱迪生氏病；青铜色皮病
adenoma	[ˌædəˈnəʊmə] 腺瘤
aldosteronism	[ɔːldʌstərəʊˈnɪzəm] 醛甾酮症，醛甾酮增多症
cretinism	[ˈkretɪnɪzəm] 白痴病
Cushing's syndrome	库欣综合征
diabetes insipidus	尿崩症
diuresis	[ˌdaɪjʊəˈriːsɪs] 多尿；利尿
dwarfism	[ˈdwɔːfɪzəm] 侏儒症
exophthalmos	[ˌeksɒfˈθælməs] 眼球突出症
glioma of pineal gland	松果体胶质瘤

第一部分　医学英语

续表

内分泌系统病理术语	中文释义
glucosuria	[ˌgluːkəʊˈsjʊərɪə] 糖尿病
goiter	[ˈɡɔɪtər] 甲状腺肿
hypercalcemia	[haɪpəkælˈsiːmɪə] 血钙过多
hyperkalemia	[haɪpəkəˈliːmɪə] 血钾过多；高钾
hyperparathyroidism	[haɪpəpærəˈθaɪrɒɪdɪzəm] 甲状旁腺功能亢进
hyperthyroidism	[ˌhaɪpəˈθaɪrɒɪdɪzəm] 甲状腺功能亢进
hypogonadism	[haɪpəʊˈɡɒnædɪzəm] 性腺机能减退
hyponatremia	[haɪpɒnəˈtremɪə] 血钠过少
hypoparathyroidism	[haɪpəpærəˈθaɪrɒɪdɪzm] 甲状旁腺功能减退
myxedema	[ˈmɪksɪˈdiːmə] 黏液性水肿
obesity	[əʊˈbiːsətɪ] 肥胖
pheochromocytoma	[fiːəkrəʊməsaɪˈtəʊmə] 嗜铬细胞瘤
pinealoma	[pɪnɪəˈləʊmə] 松果体瘤
polydipsia	[ˌpɒlɪˈdɪpsɪə] 烦渴
polyphagia	[pɒlɪˈfeɪdʒɪə] 多食症
thyroid crisis	甲状腺危象
thyropathy	[θaɪˈrɒpəθɪ] 甲状腺病
thyroprivia	[θaɪrəʊˈprɪvɪə] 甲状腺缺乏症
virilism	[ˈvɪrəlɪzəm] 男性化现象

（三）内分泌系统检查术语

表 1-2-52　内分泌系统检查表达术语表

内分泌系统检查术语	中文释义
adrenalectomy	[ədriːnəˈlektəmɪ] 肾上腺切除术
basal metabolic rate	基础代谢率
hemithyroidectomy	[hemɪθaɪrɒɪˈdektəmɪ] 偏侧甲状腺切除术
hypophysectomy	[haɪˌpɒfɪˈsektəmɪ] 垂体切除术
insulin tolerance test	胰岛素耐量试验
isthmectomy	[ɪsˈmektəmɪ] 峡部切除术，甲状腺切除术
lobectomy	[ləʊˈbektəmɪ] 叶切除术

续表

内分泌系统检查术语	中文释义
parathyroidectomy	[ˌpærəθaɪrɒɪˈdektəmɪ] 甲状旁腺切除术
pinealectomy	[pɪnɪəˈlektəmɪ] 松果体切除术
protein-bound iodine（*PBI*）	蛋白结合碘
radioactive iodine uptake test（*RAIU*）	放射性碘吸收试验
thyroidectomy	[ˌθaɪrɒɪˈdektəmɪ] 甲状腺切除术
thyroidotomy	[θaɪrɒɪˈdɒtəmɪ] 甲状腺切开术
Triiodothyronine（*T3*） *Test*, *Thyroxine*（*T4*）*Test*, *Thyroxine-binding Globulin*（*TBG*）	三碘甲状腺原氨酸（T3）试验，甲状腺素（T4）试验，甲状腺素结合球蛋白

（四）内分泌系统药学术语

表 1-2-53　内分泌系统药学表达术语表

内分泌系统药学术语	中文释义
antihyperlipidemic	[ˈænti:haɪpəlɪpaɪdemɪk] 抗高血脂药
corticosteroid	[ˌkɔːtɪkəʊˈsterɒɪd] 皮质类固醇
insulin	[ˈɪnsjəlɪn] 胰岛素
hypoglycemic	[ˌhaɪpəʊglaɪˈsiːmɪk] 降血糖药
vasopressin	[ˌvæsəʊˈpresɪn] 后叶加压素

十、感官系统

（一）感官系统词根和组合形式

表 1-2-54　感官系统词根和组合形式表

感官系统词根/组合形式/后缀	举例
acou/o-（to hear）	*acou*stic [əˈkuːstɪk] 听觉的；声音的
ambly/o-（dull）	*ambly*opia [ˌæmblɪˈəʊpɪə] 弱视
aque-, aqu/o-（water）	*aquo*capsulitis [ɑːkwəʊkæpsəˈlaɪtɪz] 浆液性虹膜炎
aniso-（unequal）	*aniso*coria [ænɪsəʊˈkɔːrɪə] 瞳孔不等
audi/o-（to hear）	*audio*metry [ˌɔːdɪˈɒmətrɪ] 测听术
auri/o-（ear）	*auri*cle [ˈɔːrɪkl] 外耳；耳廓

续表

感官系统词根/组合形式/后缀	举例
blephar/o-（eyelid）	*blephar*optosis [blefæˈrɒptəʊsɪs] 睑下垂
choroid/o-（choroid）	*choroid*itis [kəʊrɒɪˈdaɪtɪs] 脉络膜炎
conjuctiv/o-（conjunctiva）	*conjunctiv*itis [kənˌdʒʌŋktɪˈvaɪtɪs] 结膜炎
coro-, core/o-（pupil）	*core*ctopia [kɔːrekˈtəʊpɪə] 瞳孔异位
corne-（cornea）	*corne*itis [ˌkɔːnɪˈaɪtɪs] 角膜炎
cycl/o-（round）	*cycl*itis [saɪˈklaɪtɪs] 睫状体炎
dacry/o-（tears）	*dacry*ocyst [ˈdækrɪəʊsɪst] 泪囊
irid/o-（iris in the eye）	*irid*okinesis [ɪrɪˈdəʊkɪniːsɪs] 虹膜伸缩
kerat/o-（cornea）	*kerat*ohemia [kerætəʊˈhiːmɪə] 角膜血沉着
labyrinth/o-（labyrinth）	*labyrinth*ectomy [læbəˈrɪnθəktəmɪ] 迷路切除术
lacrim/o-, lacri-（tear）	*lacrim*otomy [lækrɪˈməʊtəmɪ] 泪囊切开术
myring/o-（membrane tympani）	*myring*orupture [mɪrɪŋəʊˈrʌptʃə] 鼓膜破裂
presby/o-（old age）	*presby*cusis [prezbɪˈkjuːsɪs] 老年性耳聋
retin/o-（retina）	*retin*oschisis [retɪˈnɒskɪsɪs] 视网膜分层剥离
salping/o-（tube）	*salping*oscopy [ˈsælpɪŋəʊskəpɪ] 咽鼓管镜检查
scler/o-（sclera）	*scler*ectasia [sklɪərekˈteɪzɪə] 巩膜膨胀
staped/o-（stapes）	*staped*ectomy [ˌseɪpɪˈdektəmɪ] 镫骨切除术
tympano-（tympanum）	*tympan*itis [ˌtɪmpəˈnaɪtɪs] 中耳炎
-acousis（to hear）	an*acousis* [ænəˈkʌs] 听觉缺失
-opia, -opsia, -opsy（eye）	amet*ropia* [ˈæmetrəʊpɪə] 屈折异常
-osmia（odor）	an*osmia* [æˈnɒsmjə] 嗅觉缺失
-tropia（turning）	exo*tropia* [ˌeksəˈtrəʊpɪə] 外斜视

（二）感官系统临床和病理术语

1.感官系统炎症和感染术语

表1-2-55 感官系统炎症和感染表达术语表

感官系统炎症和感染术语	中文释义
blepharitis	[blefəˈraɪtɪs] 眼睑炎
conjunctivitis	[kənˌdʒʌŋktɪˈvaɪtɪs] 结膜炎
chorioretinitis	[kəʊrɪəʊretɪˈnaɪtɪs] 脉络视网膜炎

续表

感官系统炎症和感染术语	中文释义
choroiditis	[kəʊrɒɪˈdaɪtɪs] 脉络膜炎
dacryoadenitis	[deɪkriːəʊˈdenaɪtɪs] 泪腺炎
dacryocystitis	[deɪkriːəˈsɪstaɪtɪs] 泪囊炎，窍漏症
episcleritis	[epɪsklɪəˈraɪtɪs] 巩膜外层炎
hordeolum	[hɔːˈdiːələm] 睑腺炎；麦粒肿
iridocyclitis	[ɪrɪdəʊsɪˈklaɪtɪs] 虹膜睫状体炎
iritis	[aɪəˈraɪtɪs] 虹彩炎
keratitis	[ˌkerəˈtaɪtɪs] 角膜炎
keratoconjunctivitis	[kerətəʊkəndʒʌŋktɪˈvaɪtɪs] 角膜结膜炎
ophthalmitis	[ˌɒfθælˈmaɪtɪs] 眼炎
optic neuritis	视神经乳头炎
panophthalmitis	[pænɒfθælˈmaɪtɪs] 全眼球炎
retinitis	[ˌretɪˈnaɪtɪs] 网膜状
scleritis	[sklɪˈraɪtɪs] 巩膜炎
trachoma	[trəˈkəʊmə] 沙眼
uveitis	[ˌjuːvɪˈaɪtɪs] 眼色素层炎；葡萄膜炎
eustachitis	[juːstəˈkaɪtɪs] 咽鼓管炎
labyrinthitis	[ˌlæbərɪnˈθaɪtɪs] 内耳炎
mastoiditis	[ˌmæstɒɪˈdaɪtɪs] 乳般突起炎
myringitis	[ˌmɪrɪnˈdʒaɪtɪs] 鼓膜炎
otitis externa	外耳道炎症
otitis interna	内耳炎
otitis media	中耳炎
panotitis	全耳炎

2. 感官系统病理术语

表 1-2-56 感官系统病理表达术语表

感官系统病理术语	中文释义
achromatopsia	[əkrəʊməˈtɒpsiə] 全色盲
ageusia	[ˈɪdʒɪəzɪ] 味觉的丧失

续表

感官系统病理术语	中文释义
amblyopia	[ˌæmblɪˈəʊpɪə] 弱视
ametropia	[ˈæmetrəʊpɪə] 屈折异常；非正视眼
aniseikonia	[ænɪˈzeɪkɒnɪə] 网膜异象症
anisopia	[ænɪˈsəʊpɪə] 屈光参差，两眼视力不等
anophthalmos	[ˈænəfθælməʊz] 无眼
anosmia	[æˈnɒsmjə] 嗅觉缺失
aphakia	[æˈfeɪkjə] 少晶状体，无晶状体
astigmatism	[əˈstɪgmətɪzəm] 散光
blepharospasm	[blefærəʊsˈpæzəm] 睑痉挛，眼睑痉挛
blindness	[ˈblaɪndnəs] 失明
cataract	[ˈkætərækt] 白内障
central deafness	中枢性聋
conductive deafness	传音聋，传导性聋
corectopia	[kɔːrekˈtəʊpɪə] 瞳孔异位
cortical deafness	皮质聋，皮质性聋
cyclopia	[saɪˈkləʊpɪə] 独眼畸形
deafness	[defnəs] 聋
deuteranomaly	绿色弱
diplacusis	[dɪpləˈkjuːsɪs] 复听
diplopia	[dɪˈpləʊpɪə] 复视
enophthalmos	[ˈiːnəfθælməʊz] 眼球内陷
functional deafness	机能性聋，功能性聋
glaucoma	[glɔːˈkəʊmə] 青光眼
hemeralopia	[ˌhemərəˈləʊpɪə] 昼盲症；夜盲症
hypermetropia	[ˌhaɪpəməˈtrəʊpɪə] 远视
hyperosmia	[haɪpəˈrɒzmjə] 嗅觉过敏
hypopyon	[haɪˈpəʊpɪɒn] 眼前房积脓
labyrinthine deafness	迷路性聋
megalophthalmos	[meˈgæləfθælməʊz] 巨眼
myopia	[maɪˈəʊpɪə] 近视
nyctalopia	[ˌnɪktəˈləʊpɪə] 夜盲症

续表

感官系统病理术语	中文释义
nystagmus	[nɪsˈtægməs] 眼球震颤
ophthalmoplegia	[ˌɒfθælməˈpliːdʒə] 眼肌瘫痪；眼肌麻痹
organic deafness	器质性聋，器官性聋
otoneuralgia	[əʊtəʊnjʊəˈrældʒə] 耳神经痛
otopyorrhea	[əʊtɒpaɪəˈrɪə] 耳脓溢
otorrhagia	[əʊˈtɒrædʒə] 耳出血
otorrhea	[əʊtəˈriːə] 耳液溢；耳漏
otosclerosis	[ˌəʊtəsklɪˈrəʊsɪs] 耳硬化症
pannus	[ˈpænəs] 血管翳；角膜翳；关节翳
polycoria	[pɒlɪˈkɔːrɪə] 多瞳（畸形），多瞳症
polyotia	[pɒlɪˈəʊʃɪə] 多耳（畸形）
presbyopia	[ˌprezbɪˈəʊpɪə] 老花眼；远视
protanopia	[ˌprəʊtəˈnəʊpɪə] 红色盲
ptosis	[ˈtəʊsɪs] 下垂症
retinal detachment	视网膜脱离
retinoblastoma	[retɪnəʊblæsˈtəʊmə] 眼癌
retinopathy	[retɪˈnɒpəθɪ] 视网膜病
sensorineural deafness	感觉神经性耳聋症
strabismus	[strəˈbɪzməs] 斜视；斜视眼
synechia	[sɪˈnekɪə] 粘连
tinnitus	[ˈtɪnɪtəs] 耳鸣
tympanosclerosis	[tɪmpənəʊsklɪəˈrəʊsɪs] 鼓膜硬化
vertigo	[ˈvɜːtɪɡəʊ] 眩晕

（三）感官系统检查术语

1. 眼部检查术语

表 1-2-57　眼部检查表达术语表

眼部检查术语	中文释义
blepharorrhaphy	[blefeəˈrɒrəfɪ] 睑缝术，睑裂缝合术
blepharotomy	[blefæˈrəʊtəmɪ] 睑切开术
blepharoplasty	[bˈlefærəʊplæstɪ] 睑成形术

续表

眼部检查术语	中文释义
canthoplasty	[kænθə'plæstɪ] 眦成形术
conjunctivoplasty	[kənd'ʒʌŋktɪvəplæstaɪ] 结膜成形术
coreoplasty	[kɔːiːəʊp'læstaɪ] 瞳孔成形术
cyclodialysis	[saɪkləʊdaɪ'ælɪsɪs] 睫状体分离术
dacryocystectomy	[deɪkriːəsɪs'tektəmɪ] 泪囊摘除术，泪囊切除术
dacryocystorhinostomy	['dækrɪəʊsɪstəʊraɪ'nɒstəmɪ] 泪囊鼻腔造瘘术
dacryocystotomy	[deɪkriːəsɪs'təʊtəmɪ] 泪囊切开术
iridectomy	[ˌɪrɪdektəmɪ] 虹膜切除术
iridosclerotomy	[ɪrɪdɒsklɪə'rɒtəmɪ] 虹膜巩膜切开术，巩膜虹膜切开术
iridotomy	[ɪrɪ'dɒtəmɪ] 虹膜切开术
keratectomy	[ˌkerə'tektəmɪ] 角膜切除术
keratocentesis	[kerætə'səntɪzɪs] 角膜穿刺术
keratomileusis	['kerətəmaɪljuːsɪs] 屈光性角膜移植术
keratotomy	[ˌkerə'tɒtəmɪ] 角膜切除术
LASIK（Laser assisted in-situ keratomileusis）	准分子激光角膜原位磨镶术
ophthalmodynamometry	[ɒfθælmədaɪnə'mɒmɪtrɪ] 视网膜血管血压测定法
ophthalmoleukoscope	[ɒfθælməʊ'ljuːkəskəʊp] 偏振光色感计，色觉检测计
ophthalmoscopy	[ˌɒfθæl'mɒskəpɪ] 检眼镜检查（法）
ophthalmotonometry	[ɒfθælmə'ʊɒnəʊmɪtrɪ] 眼压测量法
peritectomy	[pɪərɪ'tektəmɪ] 球结膜环状切除术
photorefractive keratectomy（PRK）	屈光性角膜切除术
radial keratotomy（RK）	辐射状角膜切开术
refraction	[rɪ'frækʃn] 折光；折射
retinoscopy	[retɪ'nɒskəpɪ] 网膜检影法
sclerectomy	[sklɪ'rektəmɪ] 巩膜切除术
sclerostomy	[sklɪə'rɒstəmɪ] 巩膜造口术
visual field test	视野测试

2.耳部检查术语

表 1-2-58 耳部检查表达术语表

耳部检查术语	中文释义
audiometry	[ˌɔːdɪˈɒmətrɪ] 测听术；听觉测试法
conduction deafness tests	传导性耳聋的测试
fenestration	[ˌfenɪsˈtreɪʃən] 薄膜开口
incudectomy	[ɪnkjʊˈdektəmɪ] 砧骨切除术
labyrinthectomy	[læbəˈrɪnθektəmɪ] 迷路切除术
labyrinthotomy	[ˈlæbərɪnθʊtəmɪ] 迷路切开术
myringodectomy	[mɪrɪŋgəʊˈdektəmɪ] 鼓膜切除术
myringoplasty	[mɪˈrɪŋgʊplæstɪ] 鼓膜成形术
myringotomy	[mɪrɪŋˈgɒtəmɪ] 鼓膜切开术
ossiculectomy	[ɒsɪkjuːˈlektəmɪ] 听小骨切除术
otoplasty	[əʊˈtɒplæstɪ] 耳整形术，耳成形术
stapedectomy	[ˌseɪpɪˈdektəmɪ] 镫骨切除术
tympanectomy	[tiːmpæˈnektəmɪ] 鼓膜切除术
tympanolabyrinthopexy	[tɪmpənəʊleɪbɪrɪnˈθɒpeks] 鼓室迷路固定术
tympanoplasty	[ˈtɪmpənəʊplæstɪ] 中耳整复术
tympanotomy	[tɪmpəˈnɒtəmɪ] 鼓膜切开术

（四）感官系统药学术语

表 1-2-59 感官系统药学表达术语表

感官系统药学术语	中文释义
β-adrenergic blocking agent（ophthalmic）	β-肾上腺素能阻断剂（眼用）
cycloplegic	[saɪkləˈpliːdʒɪk] 睫状肌麻痹剂
miotic	[maɪˈɒtɪk] 缩瞳剂
mydriatic	[ˌmɪdrɪˈætɪk] 瞳孔放大剂；散瞳剂

第三章 医院相关英语词汇

一、医院部门及科室名称

表1-3-1 医院临床及医技科室常用术语

医院临床及医技科室	中文释义
Department of Internal Medicine	内科
Department of Surgery	外科
Department of Obstetrics and Gynecology	妇产科
Department of Pediatrics	儿科
Department of Cardiology	心内科
Department of Respiratory	呼吸科
Department of Gastroenterology, Digestive Department	消化科
Department of Nephrology	肾内科
Department of Endocrinology	内分泌科
Department of Neurology	神经内科
Department of Oncology	肿瘤科
Department of Ophthalmology	眼科
E.N.T. Department	耳鼻喉科
Department of Stomatology	口腔科
Department of Urology	泌尿科
Department of Orthopedic	骨科
Department of Traumatology	创伤科
Department of Anesthesiology	麻醉科
Department of Dermatology	皮肤科

续表

医院临床及医技科室	中文释义
Department of Infectious Diseases	传染病科
Department of Pathology	病理科
Department of Psychiatry	精神科
Department of Head & Neck	头颈外科
Department of Orthopaedic Surgery	矫形外科
Department of Cardiac Surgery	心脏外科
Department of Cerebral Surgery	脑外科
Department of Physiotherapy	理疗科
Emergency Department	急诊科
Department of Urology	泌尿外科
Department of Medical Imaging, Radiology Department	影像科/放射科
Department of Radiotherapy, Radiation therapy	放疗科
Doctor's office	医生办公室
Nurse's office	护士办公室
Pharmacy Dispensary	药房
Nutrition Department	营养科
Diet-preparation Department	配膳室
Therapeutic Department	治疗室
Blood Bank	血站
Supply Room	供应室
Disinfection Room	消毒室
Dressing Room	换药室
Mortuary	太平间
Record Room	病案室
Isolation Room	隔离室
Reception Room, Waiting Room	候诊室
Consultation Room	诊察室
Delivery Room	分娩室
Intensive Care Unit (ICU)	重症监护室
Operating Room (OR), Theater	手术室

续表

医院临床及医技科室	中文释义
Ward	病房
Out-patient Department	门诊部
In-patient Department	住院部
Nursing Department	护理部
Electrotherapy Room	电疗室
Heliotherapy Room	光疗室
Wax-therapy Room	蜡疗室
Hydrotherapy Room	水疗室
Central Laboratory	中心实验室
Clinical Laboratory	检验科
Bacteriological Laboratory	细菌检验室
Biochemical Laboratory	生化检验室
Serological Laboratory	血清检验室

表 1-3-2 医学影像科分支

影像科分支	中文释义
X-ray Room	X 线室
Computed Tomography (CT) Room	CT 室
Magnetic Resonance Imaging (MRI) Room	MRI 室，磁共振室
Nuclear Medicine	核医学
Ultrasound Room	超声室
Echocardiography	超声心动图
Interventional Radiology	介入放射
Body Imaging	身体成像
Molecular Imaging	分子影像学
Abdominal Imaging	腹部影像
Breast Imaging	乳腺影像
Mammography	乳腺 X 线摄影，钼靶

续表

影像科分支	中文释义
Musculoskeletal Imaging	骨肌影像
Neuroradiology	神经影像
Vascular and Interventional Radiology	血管和介入放射
Pediatric Radiology	儿科放射
Thoracic Imaging	胸部影像
Emergency Radiology	急诊放射
Imaging Sciences	影像科学

表1-3-3 医院行政及服务部门常用术语

医院行政及服务部门	中文释义
Hospital	医院
Administrative Office	行政办公室
President's Office	院长办公室
Enquiry	导向咨询
Registration	挂号处
Admissions	入院处
Billing and Collection Departments	计费和收款部门
Medical Information Department	医疗信息科
Human Resources	人力资源部
Financial Assistance	财务部
Genetic Counseling Services	遗传咨询服务
Hospital Library	医院图书馆
Social Work	社会工作部
Volunteer Office	志愿者办公室
Scheduling Center	预约中心
Toilet	洗手间
Gift Shop	礼品部

二、医务人员名称

表 1-3-4 常用医务人员术语

医务人员	中文释义
director of the hospital	院长
physician	内科医师
surgeon	外科医师
chief physician	主任医师
associate chief physician	副主任医师
attending doctor	主治医师
resident doctor	住院医师
general practitioner	全科医师
intern doctor	实习医师
specialist	专科医师
head of the nursing department	护理部主任
head nurse	护士长
student nurse	实习护士
E.N.T.doctor	耳鼻喉科医师
ophthalmologist	眼科医师
dentist	牙科医师
orthopedist	骨科医师
dermatologist	皮肤科医师
urologist surgeon	泌尿外科医师
neurosurgeon	神经外科医师
plastic surgeon	矫形外科医师
anaesthetist	麻醉科医师
doctor for tuberculosis	结核科医师
pediatrician	儿科医师
gynecologist	妇科医师
obstetrician	产科医师
radiologist	放射科医师
doctor for infectious diseases	传染科医师

医务人员	中文释义
epidemiologist	流行病医师
dietician	营养科医师
physiotherapist	理疗科治疗师
midwife	助产士
pharmacist	药剂医师
assistant pharmacist	药剂医士
laboratory technician	检验技术员，化验员
assistant nurse	助理护士，卫生员
controller	总务科长
registrar	挂号员
cleaner	清洁员
sanitation worker	消毒员

三、诊断和治疗

表1-3-5　诊断和治疗常用术语

诊断和治疗	中文释义
inspection	望诊
inquiry	问诊
auscultation	听诊
percussion	叩诊
palpation	触诊
biopsy	活组织检查
pathological section	病理切片
endoscopy	内窥镜检查
ECG(electrocardiogram) examination	心电图检查
EEG(electroencephalogram) examination	脑电图检查
intravenous pyelography	静脉肾盂造影术
skin Test	皮肤试验
examination by centesis	穿刺检查
routine analysis of blood	血常规分析

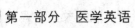

续表

诊断和治疗	中文释义
urine analysis of blood	尿常规分析
red blood cell count(RBC)	红细胞计数
white blood cell count(WBC)	白细胞计数
general check-up	全身检查
routine examination	常规检查
follow-up examination	随访检查
consultation	会诊
emergency	急诊
diagnosis	诊断
prognosis	预后
convalescence, recovery	康复
relapse	复发
treatment	治疗
prescribe	开药方
fill a prescription	配药
injecting	打针
hypodermic injection	皮下注射
intramuscular injection	肌肉注射
intravenous injection	静脉注射
inoculating	预防注射
fluid infusion	点滴注射
blood transfusion	输血
liquid medicine	药水
dose	剂量
tablet	药片
capsule	胶囊
powder	药粉
ointment	药膏（软膏）
plaster	石膏
lotion	洗剂

续表

诊断和治疗	中文释义
suppository	栓剂
analgesics	止痛药
antipyetics	退烧药
antitussive	止咳药
expectorant	祛痰药
diuretics	利尿药
hemostatic	止血药
antidiarrheal	止泻药
antipruritic	止痒药
antidote	解毒药
antirheumatic	抗风湿药
anticarcinogen	抗癌药
antibiotics	抗生素
anticoagulant	抗凝剂
cardiac tonic	强心药
vasodilator	血管舒张药
vasoconstrictor	血管收缩药
antiepileptic	抗癫痫药
antispasmodic	解痉药
sedative	镇静药
anesthetics	麻醉药
penicillin	盘尼西林
streptomycin	链霉素
gentamycin	庆大霉素
aspirin	阿司匹林
morphine	吗啡
dolantin	哌替啶
iodine	碘酒
distilled water	蒸馏水
normal saline solution	生理盐水

续表

诊断和治疗	中文释义
atropine	阿托品
hormone	激素
glucose	葡萄糖
side effect, adverse effect	副作用
operative treatment	手术疗法
major operation	大手术
minor operation	小手术
anesthesia	麻醉
general anesthesia	全身麻醉
local anesthesia	局部麻醉
excision, removal, resection	切除术
incision of abscess	脓肿切开术
tonsillectomy	扁桃体切除术
thyroidectomy	甲状腺切除术
pneumonectomy	肺切除术
mastectomy	乳房切除术
gastrectomy	胃切除术
cholecystectomy	胆囊切除术
hepalobectomy	肝叶切除术
splenectomy	脾切除术
nephrectomy	肾切除术
salpingectomy	输卵管切除术
hysterectomy	子宫切除术
hysteromyomectomy	子宫肌瘤切除术
proctectomy	直肠切除术
appendectomy	阑尾切除术
prostatectomy	前列腺切除术
tracheotomy	气管切开术
craniotomy	颅骨切开
thoracotomy	胸廓切开

续表

诊断和治疗	中文释义
laparotomy	剖腹术
amputation	截肢
fixation	固定
hot compress	热敷
cold compress	冷敷
gastric lavage	洗胃
enema	灌肠
urethral catheterication	导尿
hemostasis	止血
dressing	包扎
sew up the incision	缝合切口
remove the stitches	拆线
cardiac massage	心脏按压
artificial respiration	人工呼吸
diet	饮食
special diet	特定饮食
low protein diet	低蛋白饮食
low fat diet	低脂肪饮食
low calorie diet	低热量饮食
liquid diet	流质饮食
semi-liquid diet	半流质饮食
solid diet	固体饮食
light diet	易消化的饮食
vegetable diet	素食

四、常见疾病名称

表1-3-6 常见内科疾病术语

常见内科疾病	中文释义
acidosis	酸中毒

第一部分　医学英语

续表

常见内科疾病	中文释义
Adams-Stokes syndrome	亚—斯氏综合征
alcoholism, alcoholic intoxication	酒精中毒
alkalosis	碱中毒
anaphylaxis	过敏症
anemia	贫血
iron deficiency anemia	缺铁性贫血
megaloblastic anemia	巨幼红细胞性贫血
aplastic anemia	再生障碍性贫血
angiitis	脉管炎
angina pectoris	心绞痛
arteriosclerosis	动脉硬化
apoplexy	中风
auricular fibrillation	心房纤颤
auriculo-ventricular block	房室传导阻滞
bronchial asthma	支气管哮喘
bronchitis	支气管炎
bronchiectasis	支气管扩张
bronchopneumonia	支气管肺炎
carcinoma	癌
cardiac arrhythmia	心律失常
cardiac failure	心力衰竭
cardiomyopathy	心肌病
cirrhosis	肝硬化
coronary arteriosclerotic heart disease	冠状动脉硬化性心脏病
Crohn's disease	克罗恩病
Cushing's syndrome	库欣综合征
diabetes	糖尿病
diffuse intravascular coagulation	弥散性血管凝血
dysentery	痢疾
enteritis	肠炎

续表

常见内科疾病	中文释义
gastric ulcer	胃溃疡
gastritis	胃炎
gout	痛风
hepatitis	肝炎
Hodgkin's disease	霍奇金病
hyperlipemia	高脂血症，血脂过多
hyperparathyroidism	甲状旁腺功能亢进
hypersplenism	脾功能亢进
hypertension	高血压
hyperthyroidism	甲状腺功能亢进
hypoglycemia	低血糖
hypothyroidism	甲状腺功能减退
infective endocarditis	感染性心内膜炎
influenza	流感
leukemia	白血病
lobar pneumonia	大叶性肺炎
lymphadenitis	淋巴结炎
lymphoma	淋巴瘤
malaria	疟疾
malnutrition	营养不良
measles	麻疹
myeloma	骨髓瘤
myocardial infarction	心肌梗死
myocarditis	心肌炎
nephritis	肾炎
nephritic syndrome	肾病综合征
obstructive pulmonary emphysema	阻塞性肺气肿
pancreatitis	胰腺炎
peptic ulcer	消化性溃疡
peritonitis	腹膜炎

续表

常见内科疾病	中文释义
pleuritis	胸膜炎
pneumonia	肺炎
pneumothorax	气胸
purpura	紫癜
allergic purpura	过敏性紫癜
thrombocytolytic purpura	血小板减少性紫癜
pyelonephritis	肾盂肾炎
renal failure	肾功能衰竭
rheumatic fever	风湿病
rheumatoid arthritis	类风湿性关节炎
scarlet fever	猩红热
septicemia	败血症
syphilis	梅毒
tachycardia	心动过速
tumour	肿瘤
typhoid	伤寒
ulcerative colitis	溃疡性结肠炎
upper gastrointestinal hemorrhage	上消化道出血

表1-3-7 常见神经科疾病

常见神经科疾病	中文释义
brain abscess	脑脓肿
cerebral embolism	脑栓塞
cerebral infarction	脑梗死
cerebral thrombosis	脑血栓
cerebral hemorrhage	脑出血
concussion of brain	脑震荡
craniocerebral injury	颅脑损伤
epilepsy	癫痫
intracranial tumour	颅内肿瘤

续表

常见神经科疾病	中文释义
intracranial hematoma	颅内血肿
meningitis	脑膜炎
migraine	偏头痛
neurasthenia	神经衰弱
neurosis	神经官能症
paranoid psychosis	偏执性精神病
Parkinson's disease	帕金森综合征
psychosis	精神病
schizophrenia	精神分裂症

表 1-3-8 常见外科疾病

常见外科疾病	中文释义
abdominal external hernia	腹外疝
acute diffuse peritonitis	急性弥漫性腹膜炎
acute mastitis	急性乳腺炎
acute pancreatitis	急性胰腺炎
acute perforation of gastro-duodenal ulcer	急性胃十二指肠溃疡穿孔
acute pyelonephritis	急性肾盂肾炎
anal fissure	肛裂
anal fistula	肛瘘
angioma	血管瘤
appendicitis	阑尾炎
bleeding of gastro-duodenal ulcer	胃十二指肠溃疡出血
bone tumour	骨肿瘤
breast adenoma	乳房腺瘤
burn	烧伤
cancer of breast	乳腺癌
carbuncle	痈
carcinoma of colon	结肠炎
carcinoma of esophagus	食管癌

续表

常见外科疾病	中文释义
carcinoma of gallbladder	胆囊癌
carcinoma of rectum	直肠癌
carcinoma of stomach	胃癌
cholecystitis	胆囊炎
cervical spondylosis	颈椎病
choledochitis	胆管炎
cholelithiasis	胆石症
chondroma	软骨瘤
dislocation of joint	关节脱位
erysipelas	丹毒
fracture	骨折
furuncle	疖
hemorrhoid	痔
hemothorax	血胸
hypertrophy of prostate	前列腺肥大
intestinal obstruction	肠梗阻
intestinal tuberculosis	肠结核
lipoma	脂肪瘤
lithangiuria	尿路结石
liver abscess	肝脓肿
melanoma	黑色素瘤
osseous tuberculosis	骨结核
osteoclastoma	骨巨细胞瘤
osteoporosis	骨质疏松症
osteosarcoma	骨肉瘤
Paget's disease	佩吉特病
perianorectal abscess	肛管直肠周围脓肿
phlegmon	蜂窝织炎
portal hypertension	门静脉高压
prostatitis	前列腺炎

续表

常见外科疾病	中文释义
protrusion of intervertebral disc	椎间盘突出
purulent arthritis	化脓性关节炎
pyogenic ostcomyclitis	化脓性骨髓炎
pyothorax	脓胸
rectal polyp	直肠息肉
rheumatoid arthritis	类风湿性关节炎
rupture of spleen	脾破裂
scapulohumeral periarthritis	肩周炎
tenosynovitis	腱鞘炎
tetanus	破伤风
thromboangiitis	血栓性脉管炎
thyroid adenocarcinoma	甲状腺腺癌
thyroid adenoma	甲状腺腺瘤
trauma	创伤
urinary infection	泌尿系感染
varicose vein of lower limb	下肢静脉曲张

表1-3-9 常见儿科疾病

常见儿科疾病术语	中文释义
acute military tuberculosis of the lung	急性粟粒性肺结核
acute necrotic enteritis	急性坏死性结肠炎
anaphylactic purpura	过敏性紫癜
ancylostomiasis	钩虫病
ascariasis	蛔虫病
asphyxia of the newborn	新生儿窒息
atrial septal defect	房间隔缺损
ventricular septal defect	室间隔缺损
patent ductus arteriosis	动脉导管未闭
tetralogy of Fallot	法洛四联症
birth injury	产伤

续表

常见儿科疾病术语	中文释义
cephalhematoma	头颅血肿
cerebral palsy	脑性瘫痪
congenital torticollis	先天性斜颈
convulsion	惊厥
Down's syndrome	唐氏综合征
glomerulonephritis	肾小球肾炎
hemophilia	血友病
infantile diarrhea	婴儿腹泻
intracranial hemorrhage of the newborn	新生儿颅内出血
intussusception	肠套叠
necrotic enterocolitis of newborn	新生儿坏死性小肠结膜炎
neonatal jaundice	新生儿黄疸
nutritional iron deficiency anemia	营养性缺铁性贫血
nutritional megaloblastic anemia	营养性巨幼细胞性贫血
poliomyelitis	骨髓灰质炎
premature infant	早产儿
primary tuberculosis	原发性肺结核
progressive muscular dystrophy	进行性肌肉营养不良
pulmonary stenosis	肺动脉狭窄
purulent meningitis	化脓性脑膜炎
rickets	佝偻病
sepsis of the newborn	新生儿败血症
tetanus of the newborn	新生儿破伤风
thrush	鹅口疮，真菌性口炎
varicella	水痘
viral encephalitis	病毒性脑炎
viral myocarditis	病毒性心肌炎

表 1-3-10　常见妇产科疾病

常见妇产科疾病术语	中文释义
abortion	流产
adenomyosis	子宫内膜异位症
amniotic fluid embolism	羊水栓塞
Bartholin's cyst	巴氏腺囊肿
carcinoma of cervix	子宫颈癌
carcinoma of endometrium	子宫内膜癌
carcinoma of ovary	卵巢癌
cervicitis	宫颈炎
chorio-epithelioma	绒毛膜上皮癌
corpora luteum cyst	黄体囊肿
dystocia	难产
eclampsia	子痫
edema-proteinuria-hypertension syndrome	水肿蛋白尿高血压综合征（妊娠高血压综合征）
endometriosis	子宫内膜异位症
extrauterine pregnancy	宫外孕
hydatidiform mole	葡萄胎
hyperemesis gravidarum	妊娠剧吐
Infertility	不育症
irregular menstruation	月经失调
lochia	恶露
monilial vaginitis	念珠菌性阴道炎
multiple pregnancy	多胎妊娠
myoma of uterus	子宫肿瘤
oligohydramnios	羊水过少
ovarian tumour	卵巢肿瘤
pelvic inflammatory disease	盆腔炎
placenta previa	前置胎盘
placental abruption	胎盘早期剥离
pregnancy-hypertension syndrome	妊娠高血压综合征

第一部分 医学英语

续表

常见妇产科疾病术语	中文释义
premature birth	早产
premature rupture of membrane	胎膜早破
postpartum hemorrhage	产后出血
puerperal infection	产褥感染
rupture of uterus	子宫破裂
trichomonas vaginitis	滴虫性阴道炎
uteroplacental apoplexy	子宫胎盘卒中
vulvitis	外阴炎

表1-3-11 常见五官科疾病

常见五官科疾病	中文释义
amblyopia	弱视
amygdalitis, tonsillitis	扁桃体炎
astigmatism	散光
carcinoma of nasopharynx	鼻咽癌
carcinoma of larynx	喉癌
cataract	白内障
tinnitus	耳鸣
chalazion	霰粒肿，睑板腺囊肿
colour blindness	色盲
deflection of nasal septum	鼻中隔偏曲
deafness	聋
furuncle of nasalvestibule	鼻前庭疖
glaucoma	青光眼
heterotropia	斜视
hyperopia	远视
injury of cornea	角膜损伤
ceruminal impaction	耵聍嵌塞
iritis	虹膜炎

续表

常见五官科疾病	中文释义
keratitis	角膜炎
labyrinthitis	迷路炎，内耳炎
laryngitis	喉炎
mastoiditis	乳突炎
myopia	近视
nasal sinusitis	鼻窦炎
otitis media	中耳炎
obstruction of larynx	喉梗阻
peritonsillar abscess	扁桃体中脓肿
pharyngitis	咽炎
rhinitis	鼻炎

表 1-3-12 常见皮肤科疾病

常见皮肤科疾病	中文释义
acne	痤疮
carcinoma of skin	皮肤癌
bed sore	褥疮
decubitus ulcer	褥疮性溃疡
drug eruption	药皮疹
eczema	湿疹
herpes simplex	单纯疱疹
herpes zoster	带状疱疹
lupus erythematosus	红斑狼疮
psoriasis	牛皮癣
urticaria	荨麻疹
wart	疣

五、常见手术名称

表1-3-13 常见普外科手术

手术名称	中文释义
appendectomy (appendicectomy)	阑尾切除术
cholecystectmy	胆囊切除术
cholecystostomy	胆囊造口术
drainage of the abscess	脓肿引流
enterostomy	肠造口术
exploratory laparotomy	开腹探查术
gastrectomy	胃切除术
gastroduodenostomy	胃十二指肠吻合术
hemorrhoidectomy	痔切除术
hepaticotomy	肝管切开术
hepatectomy	肝切除术
herniorrhaphy	疝修补术
ligation of lower oesophageal veins	低位食管静脉结扎
pancreatectomy	胰切除术
portal vena cava anastomosis	门腔静脉吻合术
pyloroplasty	幽门成形术
mastectomy	乳房切除术
splenectomy	脾切除术
thyroidectomy	甲状腺切除术
thyroid lobectomy	甲状腺叶切除术
vagotomy	迷走神经切断术

表1-3-14 常见骨科手术名称

手术名称	中文释义
amputation	截肢
arthrodesis	关节固定术
curettage if bone tumor	骨瘤刮除术
excision of bone tumor	骨瘤切除术

续表

手术名称	中文释义
external fixation	外固定
fasciotomy	筋膜切开术
free skin graft	自由皮瓣移植
internal fixation	内固定
plaster cast	石膏管形
plaster splintage	石膏夹板固定
prosthetic replacement for joint	人工关节置换术
reduction of fracture	骨折复位
reduction of joint dislocation	关节脱位复位
repair if ligament	韧带修补
replantation if digit	断指再植
skeletal traction	骨牵引
tenorrhaphy	腱缝合术

表 1-3-15　常见胸心外科手术

手术名称	中文释义
aortocoronary bypass	主动脉冠状动脉分流
closed drainage of pleural cavity	胸腔闭式引流
complete intracardiac repair of Fallot's Tetralogy	法洛四联征完全修复术
dilation of aortic valular stenosis	主动脉瓣狭窄扩张术
exploratory thoracotomy	开胸探查
heart transplantation	心脏移植
heart valve replacement	心脏瓣膜置换术
ligation of patent ductus arteriosis	动脉导管未闭结扎术
lobectomy of lungs	肺叶切除
local excision of tumor of lungs	肺肿瘤局部切除术
parial esophagectomy and reconstruction of esophagus	食管部分切除、重建
atrial septal defect repair	房间隔缺损修补术
ventricular septal defect repair	室间隔缺损修补术

续表

手术名称	中文释义
valvular insufficiency repair	瓣膜关闭不全修补术
pericardiectomy	心包切除术
peicardiotomy	心包切开术
pulmonary embolectomy	肺动脉栓子切除术
resection of arterial aneurysm	动脉瘤切除术

表 1-3-16 常见泌尿外科手术

手术名称	中文释义
cystoplasty	膀胱成形术
cystostomy	膀胱造口术
nephrectomy	肾切除术
nephrostomy	肾造口术
nephrolithotomy	肾石切除术
orchiectomy	睾丸切除术
prostatectomy	前列腺切除术
renal biopsy	肾活检
renal transplantation	肾移植
urethra-lithotomy	输尿管结石切除
urethroplasty	尿道成形术
vasoligation	输精管结扎术

表 1-3-17 常见神经外科手术

手术名称	中文释义
decompression	减压术
excision of brain tumor	脑瘤切除术
exploratory craniotomy	开颅探查术
lobectomy	（脑）叶切除术
removed of intracranial hematoma	颅内血肿清除术
repair of dura defect	硬脑膜缺损修补术

表1-3-18 常见口腔科手术

手术名称	中文释义
dental prosthetics	镶牙
filling	补牙
orthodontic treatment	牙矫正术
periodontal treatment	牙周治疗
tooth extraction	拔牙

表1-3-19 常见妇产科手术

手术名称	中文释义
amniocentesis	羊膜穿刺术
cervicectomy	子宫颈切除术
cesarean section	剖宫产术剖腹产
culdocentesis	后穹隆穿刺术
dilatation of the cervix	宫颈扩张术
excision of Bartholin cyst	巴氏腺囊肿切除术
hysterectomy	子宫切除术
induction of labor	引产术
ovarian cystectomy	助产术
oophorectomy	卵巢切除术
salpingectomy	输卵管切除术
sterilization	绝育术
uterine curettage	刮宫术
vulvectomy	外阴切除术

表1-3-20 常见五官科手术

手术名称	中文释义
aspiration of cataract	白内障吸出术
closed reduction of nasal bone	鼻骨闭合复位
corneal grafting	角膜移植
enucleation of eyeball	眼球摘除术
excision of turbinates	鼻甲切除术

续表

手术名称	中文释义
extraction of intra-ocular foreign body	眼内异物摘除
laryngectomy and laryngostomy	喉切除术和喉造口术
lens extraction	晶体摘除
mastoidectomy	乳突切开术
myringotomy	鼓膜切开术
myringoplasty	鼓膜成形术
nasal polypectomy	鼻息肉切除术
septoplasty	（鼻）中隔成形术
sinusotomy	鼻窦切开术
submucous resection of nasal septum	鼻中隔黏膜下切除术
tonsillectomy	扁桃体切除术

第二部分　医学影像学基础

第一章　医学影像学发展简史

A Brief History of Radiology

With radiology being the hottest and most technologically advancing speciality, attracting the attention of many doctors, let us have a brief look at how it all began.

Radiology has been around for over a century. It all started when Wilhelm Conrad Röntgen discovered X-rays in 1895. After working for weeks in his lab experimenting on the production of "strange rays", which he referred to as "X", he asked his wife Anna Bertha to lend "a hand", the left one to be precise, which he used to produce the first X-ray image. This is now known as "Hand mit Ringen". Allegedly she exclaimed in fear "I have seen my death!" after seeing the image.

This discovery resulted in his paper "On a New Kind of Rays", earning him the first Nobel Prize in Physics in 1901.

This phenomenon sparked a great deal of interest all over the world. Within weeks of his announcement hospitals world-wide had taken the initiative to open up X-ray rooms, which gave rise to the first radiology departments. The British Röntgen Society (the first radiology society) was founded in 1897, and many further studies on X-ray usage and the effects of radiation were performed over the following years.

In the early twentieth century, it was a common goal for investigators to try to find a way to separate the superimposed shadows that were recorded when a complex structure was shown on a radiograph.

Many different methods were tried until 1921, when the Parisian physicist, André Bocage, described the basic principles of moving both the X-ray tube and the plate in synchrony while taking the image to gain a clearer image of the structure in question. This is what is known as tomography. Tomography originates from the Greek words "tomos", meaning "slice" or "section", and "graphia", meaning "description of".

In the 1960s computers were increasingly available and more powerful and in 1971, the first computed tomography (CT) scan was performed on a patient. The CT scanner was invented by Sir Godfrey Hounsfield and interestingly, at the beginning, it was not for use in medicine, but his concept was that "you can determine what was present in a box by taking a look at it from all angles".

In his workshop at the Electrical and Musical Industries (EMI, Ltd.) laboratories in Hayes, Middlesex, he worked on a computer device that was able to process hundreds of X-ray beams to formulate a 2-D image of soft tissues inside a living organism. Images were recorded on a sensor, rather than a film, and they were taken using a rotating X-ray source. These images were obtained as a series of "slices" and he was able to demonstrate the different tissue densities. It was possible to obtain 3-D volumes when the images were taken at short intervals.

He initially tested this new CT methodology using the head of a cow from a slaughterhouse before moving onto his first human patient in 1971, a woman with a suspected tumour at Atkinson Morley's Hospital in Wimbledon.

The invention of the CT scanner earned Sir Godfrey Hounsfield a

Nobel Prize in 1979 (along with Allan Cormack who came up with the underlying theoretical mathematics) as well as many other awards and recognitions. The CT scanner is recognized as one of the top revolutionary advances in medicine today, alongside the discovery of Penicillin.

Nuclear magnetic resonance (NMR), which was known as the spinning atom effect, was discovered in the late 1930s. However, it was not until 1970 that NMR was used for medical applications. In the 1960s and 1970s, scientific research was published about the diffusion, relaxation and chemical exchange of water intracellularly, eventually leading to Magnetic resonance imaging (MRI).

In 1971, an American-Armenian doctor, Raymond Damadian, published a paper in the journal Science, where he stated that NMR can detect tumours in the living body as it can distinguish tumours from normal tissue from MR relaxation times. Damadian then invented an "Apparatus" to achieve body scanning by spatially locating a tumour within the body and directing the NMR beams to specific sites of the body. He named this the focusing NMR concept (FONAR). He, along with other scientists, then performed the first human full-body scan using the FONAR scan in 1977. This image nearly took him 5 hours to acquire.

In 1973, Paul Christian Lauterbur, an American chemist and Sir Peter Mansfield, a British physicist, worked on obtaining useful magnetic resonance (MR) images taken at a much higher speeds, compared to Damadian's FONAR scanner, by varying the strength of the magnetic field and developing mathematical processes. This earned them a Nobel Prize in Physiology or Medicine that they both shared in 2003. Their work gave rise to the modern MRI scanners we use today.

Interventional Radiology (IR) came to life through the combination of the creative thinking and technical skills of diagnostic radiologists and angiogiographers. Charles Dotter, a vascular radiologist and commonly known as "The Father of Interventional Radiology", invented angioplasty. On January 16, 1964, Dotter percutaneously dilated a tight stenosis of the superficial femoral artery in an woman with painful leg ischemia and gangrene who refused leg amputation. It was a success and circulation returned to her leg. The dilated artery remained open until her death from pneumonia over two years later. This led the way for many other minimally invasive vascular procedures. Nowadays, IR is a clinically oriented speciality that offers a wide range and growing number of procedures.

The theoretical basis for ultrasound physics has been around since 1794, but it wasn't until 1942, when Dr Karl Theodore Dussik in Austria transmitted an ultrasound beam through a human skull to view the brain, that ultrasound was first used in medicine. In the mid-1950s, Ian Donald, a Professor of Midwifery at Glasgow University, became a pioneer in the application of ultrasound since he was the first to incorporate it in Obstetrics and Gynaecology. He published an article titled "Investigation of Abdominal Masses by Pulsed Ultrasound" in 1958 in the medical journal, *The Lancet*. This was a defining publication in the field of medical ultrasound.

In 1957, Ian Donald and Tom Brown, a Scottish Engineer, built the first successful ultrasound machine. It was only taken seriously after a large ovarian cyst in a female patient was diagnosed, as at first Donald's idea was ridiculed. Ultrasound was later used as a safer imaging modality for pregnant patient as X-ray use was dangerous to the foetus of a pregnant patient, as demonstrated by a research conducted by Alice Steward, a British Epidemiologist.

Radiologists needed a common means for sharing images. In the mid-1980s picture archiving and communication systems (PACS) emerged, which facilitated remote viewing of images and the prompt retrieval of images from an electronic storage.

Computer-aided diagnosis (CAD) emerged in the early 1980s. It is now being used widely in the detection and diagnosis of various abnormalities using different imaging modalities. It has become one of the most important topics of research and development in clinical radiology.

Another major advancement in radiology is artificial intelligence (AI). Early in the 1960s and 1970s, Dendral, the world's first problem-solving program, was developed. It was first intended for practitioners of organic chemistry and later provided the basis of MYCIN, a system involving one of the earliest uses of AI in medicine. AI is now becoming more mainstream with algorithms being produced to aid radiologists in the detection and characterization of pathology. AI is currently being used for many applications in radiology; for example, in speech recognition, detecting and characterizing lung nodules, characterizing liver lesions in MRI and prioritizing follow up evaluations and identifying and characterizing microcalcifications in mammograms. Currently the cutting-edge AI algorithms have a limited range of abnormalities that they can detect and require heavy tuning of parameters. As there are risks for false positives and false negatives, research is currently underway on this rapidly evolving and developing technology.

AI research is making progress

With these advancements there has been a noticeable rise in demand for radiology due to its importance in the diagnosis and management of patients. There has been pressure on limited resources due to the increase in the number of patients per radiologist. The introduction of digital radiographic techniques in conventional radiology was gradual and has been beneficial to the profession with increased image accessibility, elimination of loss of images and improved staff productivity. Images as well as their reports are now accessed within seconds throughout all hospital departments.

Ok, so what do radiologists do now?

Radiologists play a pivotal role in patient care, not only reporting medical imaging, but also performing skillful procedures to aid diagnosis and treatment, such as US and IR. Radiologists are a core part of modern multidisciplinary team meetings, reviewing imaging and contributing to the discussion of treatment plans with physicians and surgeons. Radiologists are also involved in researching new methods of incorporating advancements in technology into everyday reporting. Some centers are researching the use of AI in radiology reports, for example providing a preliminary description of findings and measurements of the lesions present.

As history has shown, radiology is a technology-heavy specialty, advancing all the time. The future of radiology will involve further advancements, and maybe technology not yet discovered, to advance medicine and help patients for many years to come.

拓展阅读

The Eclectic History of Medical Imaging

Greg Freiherr

From engineering to science, medicine and music

Physicians at Northwestern Memorial Hospital in Chicago were as stunned in 1979 by Godfrey Hounsfield's exclamation as Hounsfield was at the computed tomography (CT) image. "My word, what is that?" asked the inventor of computed tomography, who later that year would receive the Nobel Peace Prize for his invention.

Hounsfield may have been the only one in the room who didn't recognize the brain hematoma, wrote Lee F. Rogers, M.D., in his recollection of that day in 1979.1. But, in looking back, that should not have been a surprise. "The inventor of an imaging technology does just that, invents," Rogers wrote. "It is usually left for others to determine how and when this technology is best used."

In the early 1980s, early adopters of magnetic resonance imaging (MRI) took a collective leap of faith that its life-like images would reveal pathologies. It was a good but expensive gamble. The first machines cost millions of dollars each. It took years of experience to demonstrate their clinical value.

About the same time, ultrasound was "good enough" for OB/GYN but not much else. Engineers had the know-how to produce high-performance scanners, but vendors believed customers would be too stingy to pony up the necessary money. They were wrong. An engineer envisioned a better future for ultrasound. But clinicians took the chance and, eventually, proved the images were worth the price.

Diagnosticians were at the center of these early developments. But long before nuclear medicine was an imaging tool, it debuted with an "atomic cocktail." First mixed in 1946 from radioactive iodine, this cocktail cured a patient with thyroid cancer. Within a few years, clinicians discovered they could visualize the thyroid and other organs using atomic concoctions.

The eclectic story of medical imaging began, of course, much earlier, when Wilhelm Röntgen discovered the X-ray. The first to see "radiographs," however, were not physicians. Röntgen, a physicist, introduced them in January 1896 at the 50-year anniversary meeting of the Society of Physics. Their clinical potential was recognized a few weeks later with the publication in a medical journal of a radiograph showing a glass splinter lodged in the finger of a 4-year-old. The commercialization and mass production of X-ray tubes spread this technology around the globe, and within a few years radiography was recognized as a great medical advance.

While this history, certainly, is about technology, it is also about the people and how they turned ideas into medical tools. They include giants: some known, some not; some modest, some brash. Among them are four musicians, one of whom in 1966 described himself and other band members as "more popular than Jesus."

CT: From Beatlemania to Manic Slice Wars

Electric and Music Industries (EMI) may have owned the most famous recording studios in the world. Its Abbey Road Studios were the site of such Beatle hits as "Love Me Do," "Can't Buy Me Love" and "Revolution."

Signed in 1962, the Beatles generated enormous profits for EMI, profits that some speculate gave EMI the flexibility to allow Godfrey Hounsfield the freedom to invent CT.

A dearth of financial data about EMI budgets, amid estimates that the British government may have contributed substantially more than EMI, have raised questions about how much credit is actually due to the Beatles for one of the greatest advances in medical imaging.

One thing is for sure, however. Hounsfield did not invent CT on his own.

The British engineer built on decades of mathematical advances, notably the 1937 work of Polish mathematician Stefan Kaczmarz, who formulated the basis for a reconstruction method called "Algebraic Reconstruction Technique," which Hounsfield adapted for use in CT.

Independently, while at Tufts University in Boston, South African-born Allan McLeod Cormack developed a method for CT. So significant were his efforts that the Nobel committee awarded the 1979 Nobel Prize in medicine jointly to Cormack and Hounsfield.

Then there was the clinical connection. CT could not have transitioned to mainstream medical practice without the involvement of James Ambrose, M.D., a consultant radiologist at Atkinson Morley Hospital in London. Ambrose joined Hounsfield in 1971. Together they used CT prototypes built under Hounsfield's direction to look at animal and preserved human organs. In late 1971, the first clinical CT was installed at Atkinson Morley Hospital.

This machine, the EMI Mark 1, could scan only the brain. It was displayed in November 1972 at the Radiological Society of North America's (RSNA) annual meeting. At this meeting, Ambrose delivered the first clinical results from the use of a CT scanner.

Soon after, Robert S. Ledley, DDS, a dentist-turned-biomedical researcher at Georgetown University, invented a whole-body CT. By the late 1970s the modality was ubiquitous in the medical practices of developed nations around the world.

With the fundamentals of CT in place, the modality evolved, as corporate engineering teams chipped away at problems unique to this modality. One was an unexpectedly high failure rate of gantry motors onboard CTs built and installed by GE Medical Systems. The problem was initially thought to come from too little lubrication. But adding more lubricant had no effect. It was then learned that the grease lubricating the motor shaft turned to glue after long exposures to X-rays. Changing the lubricant solved the problem.

As scans covered more of the patient, X-ray tubes overheated. Philips solved this problem in the early 1990s by repurposing its Maximus Rotalix Ceramic (MRC) tube, which had been developed for cardiology and vascular X-ray systems. With no ball bearings to create friction and the use of a liquid-metal alloy as a lubricant, tube cooling was tripled and the scan time of Philips' CTs extended.

Periodically the industry leapt forward. In a radical departure from the status quo, Douglas Boyd, Ph.D., pioneered the use of electron beam tomography in the mid-1980s.

Electron beam tomography (EBT) scanners used a magnetically controlled electron beam to fire a thin circle of X-rays. Unfettered by the mechanical limitations of a conventional CT gantry, EBT systems delivered motion-free images of the heart and surrounding blood vessels. Its stratospheric price tag, north of $2 million, however, limited worldwide sales to about 150 scanners until matron, the company that commercialized

EBT, was sold to GE Medical in 2001.

In contrast, the advent of helical scanning had a profound impact on the modality. This leap, taken in 1989, made "step-and-shoot" CT scanning all but obsolete. The step-and-shoot gantry fired X-rays for a single rotation, then waited for the table to "step" the patient to the next position. Helical CT gantries rotated continuously, as the table propelled the patient through the gantry, slicing the patient into one continuous spiral. Subsecond rotations and thinner slices led to shorter scans and higher resolution images with fewer artifacts.

This advance, pioneered by Siemens' R&D director, Willi A. Kalender, Ph.D., was adopted first by the German multimodality vendor. GE soon followed suit, as did other makers of CT.

The next revolution — multislice scanning — took the CT community by storm in late 1998, when Toshiba, Siemens and GE launched proprietary versions within weeks of each other. The appearance of these machines triggered nearly a decade of heated competition among vendors to produce scanners with more and more slices per rotation. Quad-slice scanners gave way to ones that generated eight slices. In time, these were eclipsed by ones with 16 and then 32. In the mid-2000s, the industry achieved a milestone — commercial CT scanners that delivered 64 slices per rotation, marking the height of the industry's slice wars, as these scanners for the first time allowed routine cardiology applications.

MRI: Great Aspirations, Less Than Humble Beginnings

In many ways, Raymond Damadian, M.D., has been larger than life. When his MRI company Fonar was still exhibiting at the RSNA meeting, placards atop its booth attested to that. Composed of personal photos, including one of Damadian in 1988 accepting the National Medal of Technology and Innovation from President Ronald Reagan, the company founder was impossible to ignore, as GE found out, much to the chagrin of its executives and shareholders. In 1997 GE paid Fonar $128.7 million in damages and interest after a jury concluded that GE had infringed MRI patents held by Fonar.

No one, therefore, should have been surprised when Damadian launched a very public campaign against the Nobel Committee when he was not among those honored for developing MRI with the Nobel Prize in physiology or medicine in 2003. Physicists Paul Lauterbur of the University of Illinois at Urbana-Champaign, and Peter Mansfield of the University of Nottingham, won.

Ads in the Washington Post and other newspapers featured pictures of the Nobel medallion upside down and text arguing the Nobel committee had gotten it wrong. Damadian was just as forthright in interviews: "If I had never been born, there would never be MRI today," he told Nature.

How the committee made its decision will not be known publicly for a long time. Deliberations for Nobel Prizes are sealed for 50 years. A proponent of Damadian has opined, however, that "possible purported reasons for his (Damadian's) rejection have included the fact that he was a physician, not an academic scientist, his intensive lobbying for the prize, his supposedly abrasive personality and his active support of creationism."

What is not speculative is that Damadian was among the first to propose the use of nuclear magnetic resonance (NMR) to produce medical images. A 1971 paper he wrote in Science documented that cancerous and healthy tissue can be differentiated in laboratory rats using NMR.5Damadian later patented a technique to scan the body for tumors by taking a series of NMR readings from different spots. The company he founded was the first to win U.S. Food and Drug Administration (FDA) approval for an MR scanner to be sold in the United States.

Philips began exploring MRI with a pilot project launched in the mid-1970s, building a prototype that generated human images in 1978. Ironically the company was among the last to enter the U.S. marketplace, gaining FDA approval for a 1.5T system in 1986.

Damadian's Fonar was the first to market in the United States followed by Technicare (a subsidiary of Johnson & Johnson) and Picker. GE weighed in soon after, quickly becoming this country's major supplier of commercial MRI systems.

Although GE is widely known for its 1.5T Signa, which in the 1980s set the benchmark for image quality, the company experimented with a dizzying variety of field strengths, including 0.12T, 0.3T, 0.5T, 1T, 1.3T, 1.4T and 1.5T.

Various companies produced scanners at different field strengths. Bruker specialized in ones used for research, focusing on field strengths at 2.0T and above. Instrumentarium specialized in ultra-low field scanners, seeking a moderately priced alternative to high-cost MRI scanners. Diasonics produced ultra-low, low and mid-field systems that were "open" rather than cylindrical, as was typical.

In the 1990s, open mid-field systems were popular not only for their lower cost, but because they addressed patient complaints about claustrophobia. Hitachi rose to prominence with its successful marketing in the United States of Airis, a family of open scanners that operated at 0.3T. By the end of the decade, every major MRI vendor offered at least one open design.

Today, demand for open mid-field systems has all but evaporated. Two manufacturers — Philips and Hitachi — continue to make a high-field open product, Philips Panorama at 1.0T and Hitachi's Oasis at 1.2T. Quenching demand for open systems has been short- and wide-bore cylindrical products.

The new high-field standard is 3.0T; the workhorse is 1.5T. The latest major development in MRI is its hybridization with positron emission tomography (PET), a modality that more than a decade earlier combined with CT.

Molecular Imaging: Splitting the Atom, Combining Modalities

In the Atomic Age that followed World War II, peaceful uses for splitting the atom seemed reasonable. Nuclear energy was supposed to be the source of unlimited achievement in the post-war era, fueling not only terrestrial power plants but interstellar spacecraft, airplanes and even cars. Atomic bombs would clear ground for new roads and frack open natural gas reserves. Lost golf balls would be a thing of the past, as radioactive shells would reveal their presence no matter how thick the rough.

It was in this context of unfettered optimism that the American public first learned in 1946 that an "atomic cocktail" had cured thyroid cancer. The thyroid had absorbed radioactive iodine that killed the cancer.

Later in the 1950s, this weapon of "mass" destruction would be used in low doses to measure the function of the thyroid and identify disease in this gland. In the decades ahead, other radioactive elements would be used to trace metabolic processes.

Nuclear medicine blossomed in the 1960s, uncovering cancer hot spots in the lungs. By the next decade it was visualizing hot spots throughout the body — in the liver and spleen, brain and GI tract. In 1971, the American Medical Association formally recognized nuclear medicine as a specialty. Its radiotracers were used commonly to evaluate heart function, blood clots in the lungs, bone pain, infection, liver, kidney and bladder function, even orthopedic injury.

Nuclear medicine is typically seen as a development of the Atomic Age, but its beginnings go back much further to the discovery of radioactivity by Antoine Henri Becquerel, Marie Curie and her husband, Pierre. All three shared the Nobel Prize in physics in 1903 for their work.

In 1935, Jean Frédéric Joliot-Curie and Irène Joliot-Curie shared the Nobel Prize in chemistry for their synthesis of new radioactive elements. The radioactive iodine they synthesized for the atomic cocktail of 1946 was later used to image the thyroid gland, quantify thyroid function and treat patients for hyperthyroidism.

Following this was the discovery in 1937 of technetium-99m by Carlo

Perrier and Emilio Segre. This element, found in a sample of molybdenum bombarded by deuterons, was the first element artificially produced. (Its origin explains its name rooted in the Greek technetos, meaning artificial.)

The molybdenum generator was developed about 25 years later for the supply of technetium-99m. This generator was critically important to the widespread use of technetium, as the element's six-hour half-life made long-term storage impossible.

Just as the range of radionuclides has come a long way, so have the technologies used to record them. In the beginning, scans were performed using a Geiger counter positioned near the organ of interest.

The first images were produced in 1950 using a rectilinear scanner, developed by Benedict Cassen, who became known as the father of body organ imaging. His first automated scanning device — a motorized, scintillation detector coupled to a printer — generated images of radioiodine absorbed by the thyroid gland. This type of scanner was used until the early 1970s with various radiopharmaceuticals to visualize organs throughout the body.

Later in the 1950s, Hal O. Anger followed with the development of a scintillation camera that allowed dynamic imaging of human organs. The Anger camera, as it came to be known, was first displayed at the Society of Nuclear Medicine annual meeting in 1958, yet was not commercially produced until the early 1960s by Nuclear Chicago Corp. of Des Plaines, Ill. Siemens refined the Anger camera after acquiring Searle Analytic in 1979, which nine years earlier had purchased Nuclear Chicago. These early cameras delivered planar images. Today, single-photon emission computed tomography (SPECT) offers advantages in contrast, spatial localization and overall detection of abnormal function. The concept underlying SPECT goes back to the work of David E. Kuhl and Roy Edwards who, in the late 1950s, began taking cross-sectional images of radioisotopes in the body. Kuhl is credited with the development of SPECT, producing the first tomographic images of the human body in the mid-1970s. His work cleared the way for positron emission tomography (PET).

The development by Michael E. Phelps in 1973 of the first PET system and the synthesis several years later of 18F fluorodeoxyglucose (18F-FDG), in turn, laid the groundwork for modern PET in oncology.

Because cancer cells metabolize glucose at 10 times the rate of normal cells, malignant tumors appear as bright spots on PET scans. Similarly the commercial development of rubidium-82 in the late 1980s made myocardial perfusion imaging possible.

PET remained an elite tool throughout the 1990s. Its clinical use was hamstrung by the need for a cyclotron to produce positron emitters; the expense of acquiring and operating the cyclotron; the high cost of rubidium versus the relatively low cost of cardiac SPECT; and the capital expense of the PET scanner itself. Most limiting, however, was the lack of localization with PET.

The latter problem was solved in 1998 with the hybridization of PET with CT by David W. Townsend, Ph.D, at the University of Pittsburgh and Ron Nutt, Ph.D., then president of CTI PET systems. This flung wide open the flood gates for metabolic/anatomic imaging of cancer patients in the early 2000s. The first prototype PET/CT scanner, designed and built by CTI PET Systems in Knoxville, Tenn. (now Siemens Molecular Imaging), began operating in 1998.

Several factors ignited a manufacturing frenzy of PET/CTs a few years later. One was a regulatory mechanism for FDA approval of PET radiopharmaceuticals. This cleared the way for third-party coverage, led by Medicare. Individual sites and networks soon sprang up to supply cyclotron-produced FDG. In the wake of these developments, PET/CT quickly became the go-to modality for many types of oncologic diagnosis and follow-up.

The commercialization of SPECT/CT followed. Its adoption is only now beginning to gain momentum. Ironically this hybridization preceded PET/CT by several years. Bruce Hasegawa, Ph.D., directed the first such combination, building a prototype SPECT/CT in the early 1990s at the University of California, San Francisco.

In a further irony, nuclear medicine — once empowered by its connection to atomic energy — began laboring under this association following the nuclear calamities at Chernobyl and Three Mile Island. Molecular imaging is now the preferred moniker, as opinion leaders in this specialty seek a linkage between this term and "personalized medicine."

Radiography: X-rays Unveil a Hidden World In and Out of Medicine

Wilhelm Röntgen discovered X-rays in late 1895. But he probably was not the first to produce them.

Back then the leading inventors of the late 19th century were experimenting on cathode vacuum tubes of the type Röntgen used when he made his earth-shattering discovery. Among them: Thomas Edison, Nikola Tesla, Heinrich Hertz and William Crookes.

In fact, Röntgen was working with a vacuum tube developed by Crookes when he noticed fluorescence occurring in a nearby barium platinocyanide screen and traced the radiation back to the tube.

Soon after, with his wife's hand as a model, Röntgen demonstrated the potential of X-rays (short for "unknown" or "X" radiation) to reveal what lay beneath the skin. The medical utility of X-rays in orthopedics and surgery was soon demonstrated. Enabled by Röntgen's refusal to patent the process for making X-rays, inventors and entrepreneurs swarmed the fledgling industry.

Months after Röntgen's discovery, an Englishman, Sir Herbert Jackson, designed the first X-ray vacuum tube. American physicist Michael Pupin developed a fluorescent screen to shorten exposure time and improve the image. This would evolve eventually into the fluoroscope, just as Carl

Schleussner's use of a silver bromide-coated glass plate would lead to radiographic film.

Early X-ray tubes were succeeded by the hot cathode, high-vacuum X-ray tube. Invented in 1913 by William Coolidge, this tube would be named for its inventor. Along with a moveable grid, created by Chicago radiologist Hollis Potter, the Coolidge tube made radiography invaluable World War I.

With X-rays, surgeons dispensed with the use of probes, as they preoperatively honed in on bullets, shrapnel and other foreign bodies embedded in soldiers. In orthopedics, X-rays helped in the diagnosis of fractures.

Not all radiographs, however, were easy to read. Sometimes tissues or objects obscured what was behind them. In 1916 a French dermatologist, Andre Bocage, drafted to serve in WWI, developed a method whereby X-ray exposures taken at different angles would overcome this shortcoming. His method, called tomography, would become a standard method in radiography and the basis for CT, as well as modern day breast tomosynthesis.

In breast tomo, the X-ray tube and paired detector are driven by a motor to a series of points along an arc. Ultra low-dose exposures at each point create images that are then processed and compiled into a tomogram. Further processing creates a synthetic digital mammogram. Together these two digital images boost diagnostic confidence and reduce patient recalls, while keeping radiation exposure of the patient at the same level as mammography alone.

Whereas contemporary users of ionizing radiation assiduously avoid exposure, the pioneers of radiography often exposed their hands to gauge the penetrating power of the tubes with which they worked. Radiation burns were common to operators and patients, as exposures often went on for extended periods.

One such case involved a head radiograph taken in July 1896, for which the patient was exposed to X-rays for 14 hours. Within days, the patient's head was covered with sores; his lips were swollen, cracked and bleeding; his right ear had doubled in size; and hair on the right side of his head fell out.

Clarence Dally, a glassblower in Thomas Edison's laboratory regularly exposed to X-rays as part of his work, had both arms amputated after developing skin cancer. He died in 1904 at age 39 of metastatic carcinoma. John Hall-Edwards is notable for having taken the first X-ray during surgery and later, lost his left arm to skin cancer. Wolfram C. Fuchs, who made the first X-ray film of a brain tumor in 1899, died of cancer in 1907.

Heinrich Ernst Albers-Schönberg documented in 1904 that exposure to X-rays could damage the reproductive glands of rabbits. He was one of the first to use radiation protection devices, as well as procedures and equipment for radiation/dose assessment.

Despite such warnings, radiographic devices were widely used — and not just for medical purposes. In the 1920s, X-ray machines could be found in beauty shops across the country for the removal of unwanted facial hair on women. These machines fired X-rays directly into the cheek and upper lip. Some 20 treatments were typically involved. In 1929, the American Medical Association warned of injuries being manifested as pigmentation, wrinkling atrophy, keratoses, ulcerations, carcinoma and death.

In the 1940s and early 1950s, shoe salesmen flipped a switch and shoppers could see their toes wiggling on fluoroscopes. At their height, some 10,000 of these devices were in use at shoe stores across the United States. X-rays, emitted by a tube mounted near the floor, penetrated the shoes and feet, then struck a fluorescent screen on the other side. The image was reflected to three viewing ports at the top of a cabinet where the customer, salesman and a third person could see the results.

By 1970, the practice was heavily regulated or banned in all 50 states.

Yet one system was discovered operating in 1981 at a West Virginia store. When informed that the practice was banned by state law, the store donated the machine to the FDA.

Despite risks and misuse, there was good reason to celebrate the arrival of radiography. Properly applied, X-rays allowed noninvasive and painless disease diagnosis and therapy monitoring. They made possible medical and surgical treatment planning, and provided real-time guidance for the insertion of catheters, stents and other devices inside the body, as well as treating patients with tumors.

The widespread adoption of digital X-ray technologies at the turn of the century improved image quality thanks largely to software enhancement. It also made radiography more efficient with the elimination of film processing and the storage of electronic images.

Today digital images are sent throughout the healthcare enterprise via picture archiving and communication systems (PACS). PACS first appeared at the 1984 RSNA meeting, but were more proof of concept than product. Workstations cost hundreds of thousands of dollars. Mass storage required hundreds of optical disks. A robotic jukebox, developed in the late 1980s and capable of finding and reading a terabyte of data, was priced at more than a million dollars.

In the early 1990s, a comprehensive PACS would have cost millions, yet would have been compatible with only a minority of medical images. The American Society of Radiologic Technologists estimates that radiography examinations today represent 74 percent of all radiologic examinations performed on adults and children in the United States.

Given the cost and logistical challenges, "mini" PACS were developed. Some managed MRI and CT images. Others were specialized for nuclear medicine or ultrasound. Digital X-ray systems undercut demand for such truncated systems by producing the fodder for full-blown PACS, just as the means for storage and data transfer were becoming economically viable.

Getting to this point took a long time, however. Early attempts at digital X-ray go back to the 1970s and the use of selenium-coated metal plates. This method, called xerography, produced digital images of the breast, chest, temporomandibular joint, teeth and skull. But because dust or even moisture could degrade the image, its appeal was limited.

Various other technologies were tried. One digitized analog images using fiber optics that piped light flashes from a scintillator to charge coupled devices. These CCDs turned the flashes into electrical signals.

Another, called computed radiography (CR), used phosphor plates to record X-ray strikes. The plates were processed into images using laser light. CR systems were widely adopted in the early 2000s as a means for reducing costs related to film, as well as improving efficiency through the transmission and storage of images using PACS.

But radiography did not enter the modern digital age until the mass adoption of flat panel detectors. These were comprised of either amorphous silicon or selenium. Silicon panels recorded light flashes produced when X rays struck a scintillator. Selenium panels turned X-ray strikes directly into electrical signals.

In the mid- to late-1990s, flat panels were very expensive and their cost rose in proportion to their size. Consequently, they were first widely adopted when built into products that were relatively cost insensitive or required relatively small panels — or both. Cardiovascular X-ray systems were already high-priced; digital mammography units were new. Purchasers, therefore, were more accepting of the costs associated with flat panels. Additionally, the systems were stationary and, unlike radiography suites, required no shuffling of plates, which then were vulnerable to breakage.

Today, flat panels are available on all types of X-ray systems, even portables, which are jarred daily coming off hospital elevators and going through doorways. New flat panel designs have improved durability, as costs have come down with mass production and improved manufacturing.

Image processing has cut patient radiation exposure, while maintaining image quality. Continuing advances promise further cuts. This trend is in keeping with the ALARA principle, which calls on providers to administer doses of ionizing radiation that are "as low as reasonably achievable."

It is a far cry from the early days of radiography.

第二部分　医学影像学基础

第二章　医学影像设备

一、X 线（X-ray）

（一）X-ray machine

X-ray was discovered accidentally in 1895 by the German scientist Wilhelm Roentgen. Its most important application has been in medicine. X-ray revolutionizes the way how doctors detect diseases and injuries. For the first time, we could see bones and other structures inside the living body instead of relying on symptoms, samples or surgery.

Since the first X-ray machine was invented, various kinds of X-ray machines have been developed for diagnosing and treating many diseases. The diagnostic X-ray machine includes computed radiography (CR), digital radiography (DR) and digital subtraction angiography (DSA).

Although there are great differences among diagnostic X-ray machines for different diagnostic objectives, the fundamental structure of X-ray machines is similar, which consists of X-ray generating device, X-ray imaging device and X-ray auxiliary device.

1. Notes

(1) When directed at a target of low density, X-ray can pass through the substance uninterrupted. Higher density targets will reflect or absorb the X-ray. Thus, an X-ray image shows dark areas for soft tissue and shows light areas for bone.

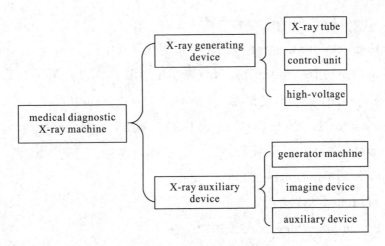

Figure 2-2-1　Component of Diagnostic X-ray Machine
图 2-2-1　诊断 X 线机组成图

当指向低密度物体时，X 射线能够不间断地穿透。密度较高的目标则会反射或吸收 X 射线。因此，在 X 射线图像中，软组织显示为暗区，而骨骼显示为亮区。

(2) The controlled filament voltage acts upon the filament of X-ray tube and heats the cathode under a certain high voltage, the temperature of cathode determines the current of X-ray tube. Thus, the filament voltage determines the radiation quantity of X-ray.

X 线管的灯丝两端加有可调节的灯丝加热电压，在一定高压下灯丝加热电压对灯丝阴极加热。灯丝温度决定了 X 射线管的电流，因此灯丝电压决定了 X 射线辐射量。

(3) As to radiation field, collimator, which is installed in the front of X-ray tube, can adjust its rotary switch to change the range of radiation field in order to reduce unnecessary radiation and grid can filter scattered radiation to improve image quality.

提及照射野，安装在 X 线管窗口的遮线器，通过调整旋转按钮改变照射野的范围以减少不必要的辐射。滤线栅则能够滤除散乱射线，以提高图像质量。

2. New Words

generate [ˈdʒenəreɪt] *vt.* 使形成，（使）产生

auxiliary [ɔːgˈzɪljərɪ] n. 辅助者设备

radiography [redɪˈɑgrəfɪ] n. [核]放射线照相术

tomography [təˈmɑgrəfɪ] n. X线断层摄影术

angiography n. 血管造影术

subtraction [səbˈtrækʃən] n. [数]减法, 减少

cathode [ˈkæθəʊd] n. 阴极

filament [ˈfɪləmənt] n. 灯丝

X-ray tube X线球管

X-ray auxiliary device X线辅助设备

high-voltage generator 高压发生器

filament voltage 灯丝电压

radiation quantity 辐射量

X-ray high-voltage generator X射线高压发生器

（二）Computed Radiography (CR)

Computed radiography (CR) belongs to digital X-ray equipment. It uses imaging plate to create a digital image. CR uses a cassette based system like analog film and is more commonly considered to be a bridge between classical radiography and the increasingly popular fully digital methods.

To use a computed radiography (CR system) – instead of the conventional film in the X-ray machine, a photo-stimulable phosphor (PSL) plate (cassette) is used for detection of X-rays. The exposed plate is scanned with helium-neon laser in the CR system scanner. The emitted light is captured by a photo-multiplier tube and converted to analogue electrical system, which is then digitised. Once digitized, it can be virtually stored and shared electronically. The image can be later printed as a film in a separate printer.

1. Notes

(1) When imaging plates are exposed to X-rays, the energy of the incoming radiation is stored in a special phosphor layer.

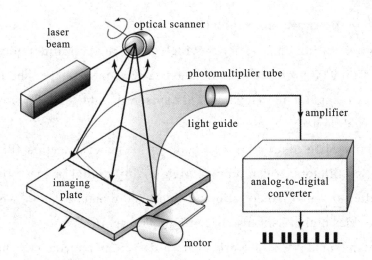

Figure 2-2-2 Identification Theory of Image Plate
图 2-2-2 IP 板读取原理图

当影像板接收到 X 线时，照射进来的辐射能被储存在一层特殊的磷光体层中。

(2) A specialized machine known as a scanner is then used to read out the latent image from the plate by stimulating it with a very finely focused laser beam.

一种被叫作扫描仪的特殊仪器被用来读出影像板中的潜影，激发潜影用聚焦很细的激光束。

(3) The imaging plate is also sensitive to other forms of radiation, including gamma rays, alpha rays, beta rays, etc. Therefore, the cassettes should be kept away from other sources of radiation.

影像板同样对其他形式的射线敏感，包括 γ 射线、α 射线、β 射线等，所以，影像板应该避光保存。

2. New Words

computed radiography 计算机 X 线摄影成像设备

imaging plate 影像板

cassette 暗盒

analog film 模拟胶片

photo-stimulable phosphor 光激励发光

helium-neon laser 氦 - 氖激光

(三) Digital Radiography (DR)

Digital radiography (DR) is widely used in the radiography field, using a digital X-ray detector to automatically acquire images and transfer them to a computer for viewing. This system is additionally capable of fixed or mobile use.

Compared to other imaging devices, flat panel detectors (FPD) are used as scintillators, It can provide high quality digital images. They can have better signal-to-noise ratio and improved dynamic range, which, in turn, provides high sensitivity for radiographic applications.

Flat panel detectors work on two different approaches, namely, indirect conversion and direct conversion. Indirect conversion flat panel detectors have a scintillator layer which converts X-ray photons to photons of visible light and utilise a photo diode matrix of amorphous silicon to subsequently convert the light photons into an electrical charge. This charge is proportional to the number and energy of X-ray photons interacting with the detector pixel and therefore the amount and density of material that has absorbed the X-rays.

Direct conversion flat panel detectors use a photo conductor like amorphous selenium (a-Se) on a multi-micro electrode plate, providing the greatest sharpness and resolution. The information of detectors is read by thin film transistors.

In the direct conversion process, when X-ray photons impact over the photo conductor, like amorphous selenium, they are directly converted to electronic signals which are amplified and digitised. As there is no scintillator, lateral spread of light photons is absent here, ensuring a sharper image. This differentiates it from indirect conversion.

1. Notes

(1) The use of digital radiography has a number of advantages. One of the most important is that the image receptors are more sensitive than film, allowing a lower patient dose.

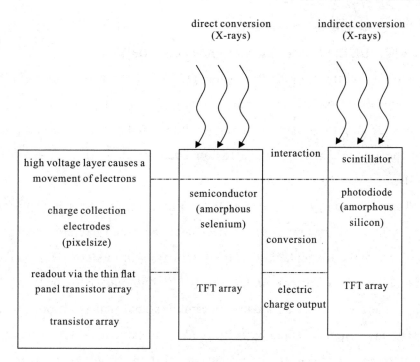

Figure 2-2-3　Transformation Process of DDR and IDR

图 2-2-3　DDR 和 IDR 转换过程比较

DR 的使用有几种优势，最重要的是影像接收装置比胶片更敏感，可以降低病人的辐射剂量。

(2) TFT array is a device that amplifies the signal then stores it as an electrical charge.

薄膜晶体管是一种可以放大并存储电信号的部件。

2. New Words

selenium [sɪˈliːnɪəm] *n.* [化学] 硒

silicon [ˈsɪlɪk(ə)n] *n.* [化学] 硅

Digital Radiography　数字 X 线成像设备

flat panel detector　平板探测器

dynamic range　动态范围

scintillator　闪烁晶体

amorphous selenium　非晶硒

photo conductor　光电导体

thin film transistor 薄膜晶体管

（四）Digital Subtraction Angiography (DSA)

Digital subtraction angiography (DSA) is a fluoroscopic technique used extensively in interventional radiology for visualizing blood vessels. Radiopaque structures such as bones are eliminated ("subtracted") digitally from the image, thus allowing for an accurate depiction of the blood vessels.

The basic components of the DSA system include the X-ray tube and X-ray generator, the image intensifier, and the video camera. Flat panel digital detectors are replacing image intensifiers in modern DSA systems. Video camera is a critical component in the imaging chain in DSA. The video camera generates an analog electronic signal that is proportional to the amount of light received by the target of the camera. At the heart of the DSA system is a digital image processing system, which acquires images from a video camera, digitizes them and stores them as digital images in the computer memory. DSA is routinely used for imaging of the abdominal, cardiac, pulmonary, carotid, intracerebral, and peripheral vessels.

1. Notes

(1) The fluoroscopy unit consists of a C-arm unit that can be rotated axially and sagittally around the floating-top table.

透视单元由 C 形臂单元组成，它可以以轴向和径向沿着活动面板检查床旋转。

(2) The distance between the X-ray tube and the image intensifier can be adjusted, as can collimation and several other parameters.

X 线球管和影像增强器之间的距离可以调节，照射野和其他几个参数也可以调节。

2. New Words

digital subtraction angiography 数字减影血管造影

image intensifer 影像增强器

interventional 介入

二、计算机断层扫描（Computed Tomography, CT）

Computed tomography (CT), sometimes called "computerized tomography" is a noninvasive medical examination or procedure that uses specialized X-ray equipment to produce cross-sectional images of the body. Each cross-sectional image represents a "slice" of the person being imaged, like the slices in a loaf of bread. These cross-sectional images are used for a variety of diagnostic and therapeutic purposes.

Unlike a conventional X-ray—which uses a fixed X-ray tube—a CT scanner uses a motorized X-ray source that rotates around the circular opening of a donut-shaped structure called a gantry. During a CT scan, the patient lies on a bed that slowly moves through the gantry while the X-ray tube rotates around the patient, shooting narrow beams of X-rays through the body. Instead of film, CT scanners use special digital X-ray detectors, which are located directly opposite the X-ray source. As the X-rays leave the patient, they are picked up by the detectors and transmitted to a computer.

Each time the X-ray source completes one full rotation, the CT computer uses sophisticated mathematical techniques to construct a 2D image slice of the patient. The thickness of the tissue represented in each image slice can vary depending on the CT machine used, but usually ranges from 1-10 millimeters. When a full slice is completed, the image is stored and the motorized bed is moved forward incrementally into the gantry. The X-ray scanning process is then repeated to produce another image slice. This process continues until the desired number of slices is collected.

Image slices can either be displayed individually or stacked together by the computer to generate a 3D image of the patient that shows the skeleton, organs, and tissues as well as any abnormalities the physician is trying to identify. This method has many advantages including the ability to rotate the 3D image in space or to view slices in succession, making it easier to find the exact place where a problem may be located.

The CT machine consists of gantry, examining table and console, most of the important components are located in the gantry, which include X-ray tube, high-voltage supply system, collimator, filter, detector, data acquistion systm and slip ring.

1. Notes

(1) Third-generation scanners have a curved array of hundreds of detectors, which are located opposite the X-ray tube and rotate as the tube rotates.

第三代扫描仪有一组曲面排列的数百个探测器，探测器位于 X- 线管对面，并且随着球管的旋转而旋转。

(2) The CT table has a wide range of horizontal movement, allowing the patient to easily move through the gantry during the scan.

CT 检查床在水平方向可大范围移动，在扫描过程中允许病人轻松地进出机架。

(3) Spiral (helical) and multislice (multidetector) CT has a dramatic effect on reducing scan time and improving image quality.

多层螺旋 CT 在缩短扫描时间、提高图像质量方面有巨大的作用。

2. New Words

fixed X-ray tube 固定阳极 X 线管

noninvasive [ˌnɒnɪnˈveɪsɪv] *adj.* 非侵入性的

cross-sectional *adj.* 断面的

gantry [ˈgæntrɪ] *n.* 机架

high-voltage supply system *n.* 高压发生器

collimator *n.* 准直器

filter *n.* 滤过器

slip ring *n.* 滑环

data acquistion systm 数据采集系统

三、磁共振成像（Magnetic Resonance Imaging, MRI）

Magnetic resonance imaging is another method available for displaying organs and systems. the phenomenon of nuclear magnetic resonance (NMR) was first described in 1946, and its early application was found in investigating the properties of matter.

The complete MRI system consists of a large bore magnet (superconducting, resistive or permanent), stable power supplies for precise magnet control, transmitter / receiver electronics for radio frequency (RF), and imaging computer and array processor with Fast Fourier Transform (FFT) hardwired for rapid computation of reconstructed images.

A magnet is essential for producing the initial conditions of nuclear alignment. A generator of radio frequency pulses is needed to perturb the processing nuclei, and an RF receiver is also necessary to detect the resulting return pulse signals from the patient.

Magnetic fields can be produced either by electromagnets or by permanent magnets. Three types exist commercially: superconducting electromagnet, resistive electromagnet and permanent magnet.

Superconductive magnets are electromagnets where the coils carrying the current are made of metals or alloys which have zero resistivity at very low temperatures. The metal alloys used are niobium - titanium, and the temperature is kept at 269 ℃ below zero by immersion in liquid helium.

Radio frequency (RF) coils produce the excitation in the static magnetic field and also pick up the emitted signal on decay. They are usually saddle-shaped and direct their field perpendicular to the direction of the main field of magnetization. The coils also collect the return signal from the patient, which is based on selection of different tissues.

The body coil is used as the transmission antenna delivering precise frequencies which determine the slice position within the coil. The NMR signal is picked up by either the same body coil or more commonly by specialized receiver coil, called surface coils, designed to cover the anatomy of interest (spine, breast, knee, etc). Surface coils are used as detectors and body coil as the transmitter.

1. Notes

(1) Magnetic Resonance Imaging (MRI) is a non-invasive imaging technology that produces three dimensional detailed anatomical images.

MRI 是一种非侵入性的成像技术，可以提供三维的精细的解剖结构图像。

(2) MRI is able to produce cross-sectional images of the body with excellent soft tissue contrast.

MRI 能够提供非常好的带软组织对比的人体断面图像。

(3) MRI scanners use strong magnetic fields and radio waves (radiofrequency energy) to make images. The signal in an MR image comes mainly from the protons in fat and water molecules in the body.

磁共振扫描仪用强磁场和射频波（射频能量）来成像。磁共振图像信号主要来自人体中脂肪和水分子中的氢质子。

2. New Words

magnet [ˈmæɡnɪt] *n.* 磁铁；[电磁] 磁体

resonance [ˈrezənəns] *n.* 共振，共鸣

coil [kɒɪl] *n.* 线圈

permanent [ˈpɜːm(ə)nənt] *adj.* 永久的，永恒的

alignment [əˈlaɪnm(ə)nt] *n.* 队列，排成直线

electromagnet [ɪˌlektrə(ʊ)ˈmæɡnɪt] *n.* 电磁体，[电] 电磁铁

resistivity [ˌrɪzɪˈstɪvɪtɪ] *n.* [电] 电阻率，抵抗力

niobium [naɪˈəʊbɪəm] *n.* [化学] 铌

titanium [taɪˈteɪnɪəm] *n.* [化学] 钛

helium [ˈhiːlɪəm] *n.* [化学] 氦

magnetization [ˌmæɡnɪtaɪˈzeɪʃən] *n.* 磁化，磁化强度

antenna [ænˈtenə] *n.* [电讯] 天线

bore [bɔ:] *n.* 孔

conduct [ˈkɒndʌkt] *vi.* 导电

nucleus [ˈnju:klɪəs] *n.* 原子核

saddle [ˈsædl] *n.* 鞍形架，鞍状物

permanent magnet 永磁型磁场

zero resistivity 零电阻

magnetic field uniformity 磁场的均匀性

radio frequency coils 射频线圈

gradient coils 梯度线圈

body coils 体线圈

surface coils 表面线圈

四、医学超声设备（Medical Ultrasonic Equipment）

Medical ultrasound (diagnostic sonography or ultrasonography) is a diagnostic imaging technique based on the application of ultrasound. It is used to see internal body structures such as tendos, muscles, joints, vessels and internal organs. Its aim is often to find a source of a disease or to exclude any pathology.

 Transducer probes, which send ultrasonic sound waves (above the range of human hearing) created within thanks to piezoelectric effect, and receive them to convert the echoes into electrical signals. They come in many shapes and sizes which determine the field of view, the frequency of emitted sound waves, and consequently how deep the sound waves will penetrate.

The central processing unit (CPU), which performs all computations, supplies the software, stores the processed data contains the electrical power supplies for itself and the transducer probe.

Transducer pulse controls, which change the amplitude, frequency, and duration of the pulses.

Monitor, which displays the reconstructed image.

第二部分　医学影像学基础

Keyboard/Cursor, which help to input data, control the screen and take measurements from the monitor.

1. Notes

(1) The main circuits of B-mode ultrasonic diagnostic instrument contains ultrasonic transmitting control circuit, signal receiving and pre-processing circuit, signal digitalizing and storing circuit, control circuit and power circuit.

B型超声诊断仪的主要电路包括超声发射控制电路、信号接收与预处理电路、信号数字化处理与贮存电路、系统控制电路和电源电路。

(2) Except for strong function of signal pre-processing, signal receiving and pre-processing circuit also is in charge of amplifying echo signal and demodulation so as to make it have enough video output power and send it to digital scan converter circuit.

信号接收和预处理电路具有较强的信号预处理功能，同时负责对回波信号的放大和检波任务，使之具有足够的视频输出功率，最后送往数字扫描变换器电路。

2. New Words

probe [prəʊb] *n.* 探头

ultrasound [ˈʌltrəsaʊnd] *n.* 超声

sonography [səˈnɒɡrəfɪ] *n.* 超声波扫描术；超声波检查法

tendo [ˈtendəʊ] *n.* [解剖] 腱

muscle [ˈmʌs(ə)l] *n.* 肌肉；力量

joints [dʒɒɪnts] *n.* [解剖] 关节

vessel [ˈves(ə)l] *n.* [组织] 脉管，血管

organ [ˈɔːɡ(ə)n] *n.* [生物] 器官

piezoelectric [piːˌeɪzəʊɪˈlektrɪk] *adj.* [电] 压电的

reconstructed *adj.* 重建的

transducer [trænzˈdjuːsə] *n.* [电子] 换能器

第三章 医学影像检查技术

一、分类

（一）X线（X-Ray Studies）

X-ray imaging is used in a variety of ways to detect pathologic conditions. Digital radiography is a form of X-ray imaging in which digital X-ray sensors are used instead of traditional photographic film. Thus images can be enhanced and transferred easily, and less radiation can be used than in conventional radiology. The most common use of diagnostic X-ray studies is in dental practice, to locate cavities in teeth (dental caries). Other areas examined include the digestive, nervous, reproductive, and endocrine systems and the chest and bones. Mammography uses low-dose x-rays to visualize breast tissue. Some special diagnostic X-ray techniques are described next.

Computed Tomography (CT). The CT scan, sometimes called "CAT scan" (because the technique originally was known as "computerized axial tomography"), is made by beaming X-rays at multiple angles through a section of the patient's body. The absorption of all of these X-rays, after they pass through the body, is detected and used by a computer to create multiple views, especially cross-sectional images. The ability of a CT scanner to detect abnormalities (the sensitivity of the scanner) is increased with the use of iodine-containing contrast agents, which outline blood vessels and confer additional density to soft tissues.

CT scanners are highly sensitive in detecting disease in bones and can actually provide images of internal organs that are impossible to visualize with ordinary X-ray technique. New ultrafast CT scanners can produce a three-dimensional (3D) image of a beating heart and surrounding blood vessels. State-of-the-art scanners produce images in 64, 128, 256, and 320 slices and are called multidetector CT or MDCT scanners.

Contrast Studies. In x-ray film, the natural differences in the density of body tissues (e.g., from air in lung or from calcium in bone) produce contrasting shadow images on the X-ray film; however, when x-rays pass through two adjacent body parts composed of substances of the same density (e.g., different digestive organs in the abdomen), their images cannot be distinguished from one another on the film or on the screen. It is necessary, then, to inject a contrast medium into the structure or fluid to be visualized so that a specific part, organ, tube, or liquid can be visualized as a negative imprint on the dense contrast agent.

The following are contrast materials used in diagnostic radiologic studies: (Barium Sulfate. Barium sulfate is a radiopaque medium that is mixed in water and used for examination of the upper and lower GI (gastrointestinal) tract. An upper GI series (UGI) involves oral ingestion of barium sulfate so that the esophagus, stomach, and duodenum can be visualized. A small bowel follow-through (SBFT) series traces the passage of barium in a sequential manner as it passes through the small intestine. A barium enema (BE) study is a lower GI series that opacities the lumen (passageway) of the large intestine using an enema containing barium sulfate. This test has largely been replaced by endoscopy, which allows visualization of the inside of the bowel.

A double-contrast study uses both a radiopaque and a radiolucent contrast medium. For example, the walls of the stomach or intestine are coated with barium and the lumen is filled with air. These radiographs show the pattern of mucosal ridges.

Iodine Compounds. Radiopaque fluids containing up to 50% iodine are used in the following tests:

Angiography

X-ray image (angiogram) of blood vessels and heart chambers is obtained after contrast is injected through a catheter into the appropriate blood vessel or heart chamber. In clinical practice, the terms angiogram and arteriogram are used interchangeably. Coronary angiography, which determines the degree of obstruction of the arteries that supply blood to the heart.

Cholangiography

X-ray imaging after injection of contrast into bile ducts. This is typically accomplished by injecting contrast directly into the common bile duct via a procedure called endoscopic retrograde cholangiopancreatography (ERCP) or after surgery of the gallbladder or biliary tract (intraoperative cholangiography). An alternative route for injection of contrast is via a needle through the skin and into the liver. This is percutaneous transhepatic cholangiography.

Interventional Radiology. Interventional radiologists perform invasive procedures (therapeutic or diagnostic) usually under CT guidance or fluoroscopy. Fluoroscopy is the use of X-rays and a fluorescent screen to produce real-time video images. Procedures include percutaneous biopsy, placement of drainage catheters, drainage of abscesses, occlusion of bleeding vessels, and catheter instillation of antibiotics or chemotherapy agents. In addition, interventional radiologists perform radiofrequency ablation (removal) of tumors and tissues (liver, kidney, adrenals). Neurointerventional radiologists perform endovascular procedures including intracranial thrombolysis, head, neck, and intracranial tumor embolizations, extracranial angioplasty and stenting. They also perform nonvascular procedures, such as intervertebral facet injections, nerve root blocks, and vertebroplasties. Vascular interventional radiologists perform laser treatments for varicose veins and uterine fibroid embolization.

（二）超声影像（Ultrasound Imaging）

Ultrasound imaging, or ultrasonography, uses high-frequency inaudible sound waves that bounce off body tissues and are then recorded to give information about the anatomy of an internal organ. An instrument called a transducer or probe is placed near or on the skin, which is covered with a thin coating of gel to ensure good transmission of sound waves. The transducer emits sound waves in short, repetitive pulses. The ultrasound waves move through body tissues and detect interfaces between tissues of different densities. An echo reflection of the sound waves is formed as the waves hit the various body tissues and bounce back to the transducer.

These ultrasonic echoes are then recorded as a composite picture of the area of the body over which the instrument has passed. The record produced by ultrasound is called a sonogram.

Ultrasound imaging is used as a diagnostic tool not only by radiologists but also by neurosurgeons and ophthalmologists to detect intracranial and ophthalmic lesions. Cardiologists use ultrasound techniques to detect heart valve and blood vessel disorders (echocardiography), and gastroenterologists use it to locate abdominal masses outside the digestive organs. Similarly, pulmonologists use ultrasound procedures for locating and sampling lesions outside the bronchial tubes. Obstetricians and gynecologists use ultrasound imaging to differentiate single from multiple pregnancies, as well as to help in performing amniocentesis. Other uses are to image benign and malignant tumors and determine the size and development of the fetus. Measurements of the head, abdomen, and femur are made from ultrasound images obtained in various fetal planes.

Ultrasound imaging has several advantages in that the sound waves are not ionizing and do not injure tissues at the energy ranges used for diagnostic purposes. Because water is an excellent conductor of the ultrasound beams, patients are requested to drink large quantities of water before examination so that the urinary bladder will be distended, allowing better viewing of pelvic and abdominal organs.

Two ultrasound techniques, Doppler ultrasound and color flow imaging, make it possible to record blood flow velocity (speed). These techniques are used to image major blood vessels to detect obstructions caused by atherosclerotic plaques in patients at risk for stroke.

Ultrasonography is used in interventional radiology to guide needle biopsy for the puncture of cysts, for placing needles during amniocentesis, and for inserting radioactive seeds into the prostate (brachytherapy). In endoscopic ultrasonography, a small ultrasound transducer is attached to the tip of an endoscope that is inserted into the body. This technique is used by gastroenterologists and pulmonologists to obtain high-quality and accurate detailed images of the digestive and respiratory systems.

（三）磁共振影像（Magnetic Resonance Imaging）

Magnetic resonance imaging (MRI) uses magnetic fields and radiowaves rather than X-rays. Hydrogen protons are aligned and synchronized by placing the body in a strong magnetic field. Then the hydrogen molecules relax when the magnetic field is shut down. The rates of alignment and relaxation vary from one tissue to the next, producing a sharply defined picture. Because bone is virtually devoid of water, it does not image well on MRI. The MR technique produces sagittal, coronal (frontal), and axial (cross-sectional) images.

MRI examinations are performed with and without contrast. The contrast agent most commonly used is gadolinium (Gd). As iodine contrast does with CT, gadolinium enhances vessels and tissues, increases the sensitivity for lesion detection, and helps differentiate between normal and abnormal tissues and structures. MRI provides excellent soft tissue images, detecting edema in the brain, providing direct imaging of the spinal cord, detecting tumors in the chest and abdomen, and visualizing the cardiovascular system.

MRI is contraindicated for patients with pacemakers or metallic implants because the powerful magnet can alter position and functioning of such devices. However, the Food and Drug Administration (FDA) has recently approved new pacemakers that can be safely used with MRI. The sounds (loud tapping) heard during the test are caused by the pulsing of the magnetic field as the device scans the body.

MRI 与 CT 扫描对比（MRI versus CT Scanning）

Why do doctors choose MRI or CT scanning? Differences in use depend on the part of the body viewed. In general, CT is useful for visualizing bony structures and solid masses of the chest and abdomen, whereas MRI is better at giving detail in soft tissues that have more water molecules.

CT：① Bones；② Chest lesions and pneumonia；③ Bleeding in the brain from head trauma and ruptured arteries.

MRI: ① spinal cord and brain tumors；② joints, tendons, and ligaments；③ liver masses；④ head and neck lesions.

X 线体位（X-ray Positioning）

In order to take the best picture of the part of the body being radiographed, the patient, detector, and x-ray tube must be positioned in the most favorable alignment possible. Radiologists use special terms to refer to the direction of travel of the x-ray through the patient. X-ray Terms describing the direction of the x-ray beam follow and are illustrated below:

(1) Posteroanterior (PA) view In this most commonly requested chest x-ray view, x-rays travel from a posteriorly placed source to an anteriorly placed detector.

(2) Anteroposterior (AP) view X-rays travel from an anteriorly placed source to a posteriorly placed detector.

(3) Lateral view In a left lateral view, x-rays travel from a source located to the right of the patient to a detector placed to the left of the patient.

(4) Oblique view X-rays travel in a slanting direction at an angle from the perpendicular plane. Oblique views show regions or structures ordinarily hidden and superimposed in routine PA and AP views.

The following terms are used to describe the position of the patient or part of the body in the X-ray examination:

abduction	Movement away from the midline of the body.
adduction	Movement toward the midline of the body.
eversion	Turning outward.
extension	Lengthening or straightening a flexed limb.
flexion	Bending a part of the body.
inversion	Turning inward.
lateral decubitus	Lying down on the side (with the X-ray beam horizontally positioned).
prone	Lying on the belly (face down).
recumbent	Lying down (may be prone or supine).
supine	Lying on the back (face up).

（四）核医学（Nuclear Medicine）

1. 放射性和放射性核素（Radioactivity and Radionuclides）

The spontaneous emission of energy in the form of particles or rays coming from the interior of a substance is called radioactivity. A radionuclide (or radioisotope) is a substance that gives off high-energy particles or rays as it disintegrates. Radionuclides are produced in either a nuclear reactor or a charged-particle accelerator (cyclotron) or by irradiating stable substances, causing disruption and instability. Half-life is the time required for a radioactive substance (radionuclide) to lose half of its radioactivity by disintegration. Knowledge of a radionuclide's half-life is important in determining how long the radioactive substance will emit radioactivity when in the body. The half-life must be long enough to allow for diagnostic imaging but as short as possible to minimize patient exposure to radiation.

Radionuclides emit three types of radioactivity: alpha particles, beta particles, and gamma rays. Gamma rays, which have greater penetrating ability than alpha and beta particles, and more ionizing power, are especially useful to physicians in both the diagnosis and the treatment of disease. Technetium-99m (Tc-99m) is essentially a pure gamma emitter with a half-life of 6 hours. Its properties make it the most frequently used radionuclide in diagnostic imaging.

2. 核医学检查方法：体内诊断和体外诊断（Nuclear Medicine Tests: In Vitro And In Vivo Procedures）

Nuclear medicine physicians use two types of tests in the diagnosis of disease: in vitro (in the test tube) procedures and in vivo (in the body) procedures. In vitro procedures involve analysis of blood and urine specimens using radioactive chemicals. For example, a radioimmunoassay (RIA) is an in vitro procedure that combines the use of radioactive chemicals and antibodies to detect hormones and drugs in a patient's blood. The test allows the detection of minute amounts of substances or compounds. RIA is used to monitor the amount of digitalis, a drug used to treat heart disease, in a patient's bloodstream and can detect hypothyroidism in newborn infants.

In vivo tests trace the amounts of radioactive substances within the body. They are given directly to the patient to evaluate the function of an organ or to image it. For example, in tracer studies a specific radionuclide is incorporated into a chemical substance and administered to a patient. The combination of the radionuclide and a drug or chemical is called a radiopharmaceutical (or radiolabeled compound). Each radiopharmaceutical is designed to concentrate in a certain organ. The organ can then be imaged using the radiation given off by the radionuclide.

A sensitive, external detection instrument called a gamma camera is used to determine the distribution and localization of the radiopharmaceutical in various organs, tissues, and fluids. The amount of radiopharmaceutical at a given location is proportional to the rate at which the gamma rays are emitted. Nuclear medicine studies depict the physiologic behavior (how the organ works) rather than the specific anatomy of an organ.

The procedure of making an image by tracking the distribution of radioactive substance in the body is radionuclide scanning. Uptake refers to the rate of absorption of the radiopharmaceutical into an organ or tissue.

Radiopharmaceuticals are administered by different routes to obtain a scan of a specific organ in the body. For example, in the case of a lung scan, the radiopharmaceutical is given intravenously (for perfusion studies, which rely on passage of the radioactive compound through the capillaries of the lungs) or by inhalation of a gas or aerosol (for ventilation studies), which fills the air sacs (alveoli). The combination of these tests permits sensitive and specific diagnosis of clots in the lung (pulmonary emboli).

Other diagnostic procedures that use radionuclides include the following:

(1) Bone scan Technetium-99m (Tc-99m) is used to label phosphate substances and then is injected intravenously. The phosphate compound is taken up preferentially by bone, and the skeleton is imaged in 2 or 3 hours. Waiting 2 to 3 hours allows much of the radiopharmaceutical to be excreted in urine and allows for better visualization of the radioactive material remaining in the skeleton. The scan detects infection, inflammation, or tumors involving the skeleton, which appear as areas of high uptake ("hot spots") on the scan.

(2) Lymphoscintigraphy This type of nuclear medicine imaging provides pictures (scintigrams) of the lymphatic system. A radiotracer (radioactive isotope) is injected under the skin or deeper using a small needle. A gamma camera then takes a series of images of an area of the body. Physicians perform lymphoscintigraphy to identify a sentinel lymph node (the first lymph node to receive lymph drainage from a tumor), identify areas of lymph node blockage, or evaluate lymphedema (accumulation of fluid in soft tissues leading to swelling).

(3) Positron emission tomography (PET scan) This radionuclide technique produces images of the distribution of radioactivity (through emission of positrons) in a region of the body. It is similar to the CT scan, but radioisotopes are used instead of contrast and x-rays. The radionuclides are incorporated (by intravenous injection) into the tissues to be scanned, and an image is made showing where the radionuclide is or is not being metabolized. The most common radionuclide is radiolabeled fluorodeoxyglucose (18F-FDG), but others are in use. PET scanning has determined that schizophrenics do not metabolize glucose equally in all parts of the brain and that drug treatment can bring improvement to these regions. Areas of metabolic deficiency can be pinpointed by PET, making it helpful in diagnosing and treating other neurologic disorders such as stroke, epilepsy, and Alzheimer disease. Alternatively, areas of infection, inflammation, and tumor demonstrate increased metabolic activity, highlighted as hot spots on the PET scan.

(4) PET/CT scan This scan combines PET and CT techniques to produce a more accurate image than PET or CT alone. It is often used to detect cancer and metastases, especially to determine if the cancer is responding to treatment.

(5) Single photon emission computed tomography (SPECT) This technique involves an intravenous injection of radioactive tracer (such as Tc-99m) and the computer reconstruction of a 3D image based on a composite of many views. Clinical applications include detecting liver tumors, detecting cardiac ischemia, and evaluating bone disease of the spine.

Scintigraphy is the process of obtaining an image using a radioisotope. The term is derived from Latin scintilla, meaning spark. Bone scintigraphy is commonly called a bone scan, and lung scintigraphy is commonly called a lung scan.

(6) Technetium Tc 99m Sestamibi (Cardiolite) scan This radiopharmaceutical is injected intravenously and traced to heart muscle. An exercise tolerance test (ETT) is used with it for an ETT-MIBI scan. In a multiple gated acquisition (MUGA) scan, Tc-99m is injected intravenously to study the motion of the heart wall muscle and the ventricle's ability to eject blood (ejection fraction).

(7) Thallium scan Thallium-201 (TL-201) is injected intravenously to evaluate myocardial perfusion. A high concentration of TL-201 is present in well-perfused heart muscle cells, but infarcted or scarred myocardium does not take up any thallium, showing up as "cold spots." If the defective area is ischemic, the cold spots fill in (become "warm") on delayed images (obtained later).

(8) Thyroid scan In a thyroid scan, an iodine radionuclide, usually iodine-123 (I-123), is administered orally, and the scan reveals the size, shape, and position of the thyroid gland. Alternatively, radioactive technetium can be administered intravenously. Hyperfunctioning thyroid nodules (adenomas) accumulate higher amounts of radioactivity and are termed "hot". Thyroid carcinoma does not concentrate radioiodine well and is seen as a "cold" spot on the scan.

A radioactive iodine uptake (RAIU) study is performed to assess the function of the thyroid gland (such as hyperthyroidism). The patient is given radioactive iodine (in this case, I-131), also called radioiodine, in liquid or capsule form, and then a sensor is placed over the thyroid gland. It detects gamma rays emitted from the radioactive tracer, which is taken up by the thyroid more readily than by other tissues. Radioiodine also is used to treat hyperthyroidism, thyroid nodules, or thyroid cancer. After the patient swallows the I-131, it is absorbed into the bloodstream and then travels to the thyroid gland, where it destroys overactive thyroid tissue.

二、各种医学影像检查技术优缺点

One of the things patients may undergo is have some kind of "imaging" done on their bodies. These imaging tools help doctors scrutinize details of the ailing part of the body that are not visible to the naked eye, and pinpoint very specific areas of disease and treatment.

Wilhelm Röntgen discovered the X-ray in November 1895. Röntgen, a physicist, introduced "radiographs" in January 1896 at the 50-year anniversary meeting of the Society of Physics. A few weeks later, a medical journal acknowledged the clinical potential of "radiographs" when it published an article of a "radiograph showing a glass splinter lodged in the finger of a 4-year-old. The commercialization and mass production of X-ray tubes spread this technology around the globe, and within a few years radiography was recognized as a great medical advance."

Today, medical imaging comes in various forms and power. Below are brief descriptions of these imaging tools to help patients understand their importance, utility, advantages and disadvantages.

Plain X-ray

The X-ray as an imaging device shows images of bones, some tumors and other dense matter.

Advantages:

(1) Quick, painless, and non-invasive.

(2) Helps diagnose broken bones, some cancers and infections.

Disadvantages:

Very small risk of cancer in the future—especially for children—from exposure to ionising radiation (X-rays).

Computed Tomography (CT Scan)

The CT Scan has the ability to show detailed images inside the body, including bones, organs, tissues, and tumors.

Advantages:

(1) Quick and painless.

(2) Helps diagnose more diseases than plain X-ray.

(3) Helps pinpoint or exclude the presence of more serious problems.

(4) Helps verify the recurrence of a previously treated disease.

Disadvantages:

(1) Small increased risk of cancer in the future—especially to children—due to exposure to higher doses of ionising radiation (X-rays).

(2) May need to inject patient with a contrast medium (dye), which causes kidney problems or allergic or injection-site reactions in some people.

(3) May require anesthesia.

Magnetic Resonance Imaging (MRI)

The MRI uses magnetic fields and radio waves to show detailed images of organs, soft tissues, bones, ligaments and cartilage.

Advantages:

(1) Usually painless and non-invasive.

(2) Uses no ionising radiation.

(3) Helps diagnose a wide range of conditions.

(4) Helps provide similar information to CT Scan in some cases.

Disdvantages:

(1) Can be lengthy and noisy.

(2) Slight movements can ruin the image, requiring a re-test.

(3) Can make some people feel claustrophobic.

(4) Requires the patient to be very still, and so may need to sedate or anesthesize those who can't stay still—particularly children.

(5) May need to inject patient with a contrast medium (dye), which cause kidney problems or allergic or injection-site reactions in some

people.

(6) Sometimes can't be done on patients with special conditions such as when a heart pacemaker is present.

Nuclear Medicine Imaging Including Positron-Emission Tomography (PET)

With PET imaging, the patient is injected with, inhales, or swallows a radioactive 'tracer'. The PET scanner uses the gamma rays emitted by this material to show images of bones and organs.

Advantages:

(1) Usually painless.

(2) Helps diagnose, treat, or predict the outcome for a wide range of conditions.

(3) Unlike most other imaging types, can show how different parts of the body are working and can detect problems much earlier.

(4) Can check how far a cancer has spread and how well treatment is working.

Disadvantages:

(1) Patient will be exposed to ionising radiation (gamma-rays).

(2) The radioactive material may cause allergic or injection-site reactions in some people.

(3) May need to sedate patients who may feel claustrophobic.

Ultrasound

The Ultrasound is an imaging equipment that uses high-frequency sound waves to produce moving images of the inside of the body, including organs, soft tissues, bones, and an unborn baby, that are then projected onto a screen monitor.

Advantages:

(1) Usually safe, relatively painless, and non-invasive.

(2) Uses no ionising radiation.

(3) Does not usually require injection of a contrast medium (dye).

(4) Can help diagnose a range of conditions in different parts of the body, such as the abdomen, pelvis, blood vessels, breast, kidneys, muscles, bones and joints.

(5) Can be used to check on the health of a baby during pregnancy.

Disdvantages:

(1) Quality and interpretation of the image highly depends on the skill of the person doing the scan.

(2) Other factors can affect image quality, including the presence of air and calcified areas in the body (e.g. bones, plaques and hardened arteries), and a person's body size.

(3) In some ultrasounds, patients may need to have a special probe placed in their esophagus, rectum or vagina.

(4) Patient may need to have special preparations before the procedure such as fasting or having a full bladder.

第三部分　医学影像诊断病例及影像报告

第一章　医学影像诊断病例

Case 1: Cirrhosis with hepatocellular carcinoma

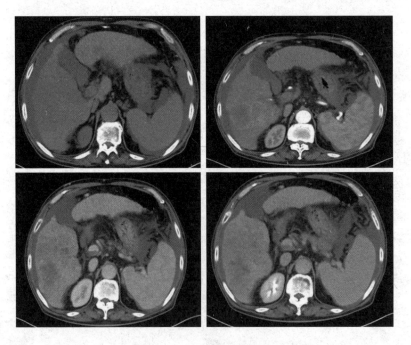

图 3-1-1　肝硬化伴肝癌

Findings

There were multiple low-density foci of different sizes in the lower segment of the right lobe of liver, with irregular shapes, unclear boundaries and uneven density. The larger ones had a cross-sectional area of about 38mmX57mm. The arterial phase of enhanced scanning is uneven and markedly enhanced, and the venous phase and delayed phase are relatively low. The liver volume decreased, the edge was uneven and wavy, the liver fissure widened, and the ratio of each lobe was out of proportion. Banded liquid density foci were seen around liver and spleen. The spleen is enlarged. The portal vein was widened, with a larger diameter of about 18mm. Enhanced scanning revealed a filling defect.The gallbladder was not enlarged, the wall was not thick, there was no positive stone shadow in the gallbladder, and the common bile duct was not dilated. The shape and position of the pancreas were not abnormal, the outline was clear, there was no abnormal density in the pancreatic parenchyma, the pancreatic duct was not dilated, and the peripancreatic fat space was clear. The spleen is small, the margin is smooth, and there is no abnormal density shadow in the spleen parenchyma. No abnormality was observed in the shape and position of both kidneys, and no obvious abnormal density shadow was observed in parenchyma of both kidneys.No abnormal enlargement of lymph nodes was observed in the retroperitoneal area.

Impression

(1) Liver cancer in the right lower lobe of liver (S5+6 segment of liver) with intrahepatic metastasis and portal vein cancer thrombus formation.

(2) Symptoms of cirrhosis, splenomegaly, ascites and portal hypertension.

病例1：肝硬化伴肝癌

征象描述

肝右叶下段多发大小不等低密度灶，形状不规整，边界欠清晰，密度欠均匀，较大者横截面积约38mm×57mm，增强扫描动脉期不均匀明显强化，静脉期、延迟期呈相对低密度。肝脏体积减小，边缘凹凸不平，呈波浪状改变，肝裂增宽，各叶比例失调；肝周、脾周见带状液体密度灶；脾脏体积增大；门静脉增宽，较大直径约18mm，增强扫描见充盈缺损。胆囊未见增大，壁不厚，胆囊内未见阳性结石影，胆总管未见扩张。胰腺形态及位置未见异常，轮廓清晰，胰腺实质内未见异常密度影，胰管未见扩张，胰周脂肪间隙清晰。脾不大，边缘光整，脾实质内未见异常密度影。双肾形态位置未见异常，双肾实质内未见明显异常密度影。腹膜后区未见异常肿大淋巴结影。

影像诊断

(1) 肝右下叶（肝S5+6段）肝癌并肝内转移、门静脉癌栓形成。

(2) 肝硬化、脾大、腹腔积液、门脉高压征象。

Case 2: Double frontotemporal parietal subdural hematomas

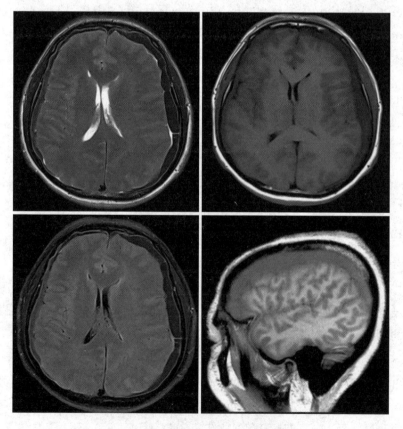

图 3-1-2　双额颞顶部硬膜下血肿

Findings

No abnormality was observed in scalp soft tissue and skull bone bone structure. The curved narrow band of long T1 short T2 signal shadow was visible under intracranial plate of the top of bilateral forehead. On the left side, limitation of adjacent cerebral sulcus was narrowed, bilateral lateral ventricles were compressed and narrowed, and midline structure shifted to the right. No obvious abnormal signal shadow was observed in the brain parenchyma at all levels. No space-occupying lesions were noticed in the sellar region and bilateral cerebellar pontine Angle.

Impression

A double frontotemporal parietal subdural hematoma (acute stage) with significant mass effect. The midline structure deviates to the right.

病例2：双额颞顶部硬膜下血肿

征象描述

头皮软组织及颅骨骨质结构未见异常，双侧额颞顶部颅内板下可见弧形窄带状长T1短T2信号影，相邻脑沟裂受限变窄，双侧侧脑室受压变窄，中线结构向右偏移。各层面脑实质内未见明显异常信号影。鞍区及双侧脑桥小脑角区未见占位性病变。

影像诊断

双额颞顶部硬膜下血肿（急性期），占位效应明显，中线结构右偏。

Case 3: A large area of acute cerebral infarction was found in the left temporal occipital lobe and basal ganglia.

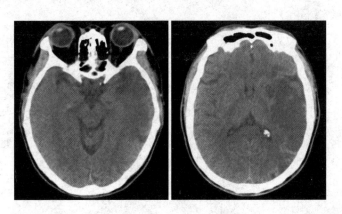

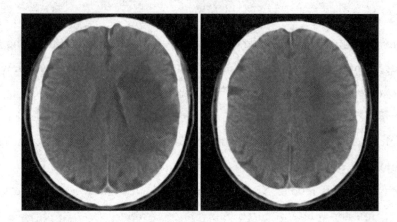

图 3-1-3　左颞枕叶及基底节区大面积急性期脑梗死

Findings

The cerebral hemispheres on both sides are symmetrical. Large low-density shadow can be seen in the left temporal, parietal, occipital lobes and the left basal ganglia. The adjacent cerebral sulcus and brain fission are narrow, and the left ventricle becomes narrow under compression. The right cerebral parenchyma and ventricle were as normal in shape, and sulci, fissure and cistern showed no widening or narrowing. No abnormal density shadow was observed in cerebellum, brainstem and medulla oblongata. The midline struciure shifts slightly to the right. No abnormality was observed in skull and soft tissue of scalp.

Impression

Large areas of acute cerebral infarction in the left temporal occipital lobe and basal ganglia area, are recommended for further examination by MR plain scan and MRA.

病例3：左颞枕叶及基底节区大面积急性期脑梗死

征象描述

两侧大脑半球对称，左侧颞、顶、枕叶及左侧基底节区可见大片低密度影，邻近脑沟、脑裂变窄，左侧脑室受压变窄。右侧脑实质、脑室形态如常，脑沟、脑裂及脑池未见增宽或变窄。小脑、脑干及延髓未见异常密度影。中线轻微向右偏移。颅骨及头皮软组织未见异常。

影像诊断

左颞枕叶及基底节区大面积急性期脑梗死,建议 MR 平扫 +MRA 进一步检查。

Case 4: Periapical lung cancer of the right upper segment

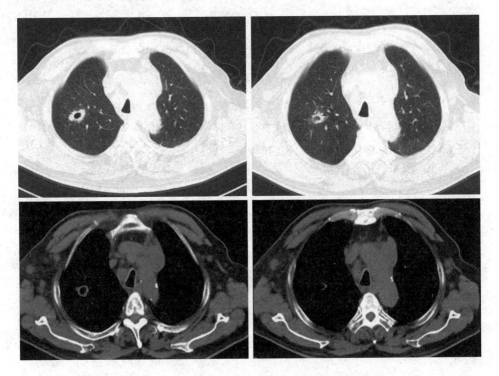

图 3-1-4　右上肺周围型肺癌伴多发淋巴结转移

Findings

The thorax on both sides is symmetrical. No abnormal changes in bone structure and soft tissue were observed.The veins of both lungs increased and thickened, and the edges were smooth and even.An irregular soft tissue nodules, about 28mm × 26mm × 16mm in size, with irregular contour and obvious lobulation, can be seen in the upper apex segment of the right lung. Air-bearing hollows can be seen inside, and the inner wall is still smooth. The margin of the nodule is irregular, and multiple long burr shadows can be seen adhering to the adjacent pleura. The trachea, bronchus and their branches were unobstructed.Bilateral hilum is not large.Multiple enlarged and fused lymph node shadows can be seen in bilateral supraclavicular fossa, mediastinum and bilateral axilla. There was no abnormality in the shape and size of the heart and the great vessels. Diffuse calcification was observed in the bilateral coronary arteries, and crescent-shaped water density shadow was observed in the pericardial cavity. No thickening of the pleura on both sides and there is no sign of pleural effusion.

Impression

(1) Right superior apical peripheral lung cancer with multiple lymphatic metastases in bilateral supraclavicular fossa, mediastinum and bilateral axilla.

(2) Pericardial effusion and coronary artery calcification.

病例4：右上肺周围型肺癌伴多发淋巴结转移

征象描述

两侧胸廓对称，骨质结构及软组织未见异常改变。两肺纹理增多、增粗，边缘尚光整。右肺上尖段可见一不规整软组织结节，大小约28mm×26mm×16mm，轮廓不规则，明显分叶；其内可见含气空洞，内壁尚光整；结节边缘不规整，可见多发长毛刺影与邻近胸膜粘连。气管、支气管及其分支通畅。两侧肺门不大。两侧锁骨上窝、纵隔内及两侧腋窝可见多发肿大、融合的淋巴结影。心脏、大血管形态、大小未见异常，两侧冠状动脉可见弥漫性钙化，心包腔内可见新月状水样密度影。两侧胸膜未见增厚，胸腔未见积液征象。

影像诊断

(1) 右肺上尖段周围型肺癌伴两侧锁骨上窝、纵膈内及两侧腋窝多发淋巴转移。

(2) 心包积液，冠状动脉钙化。

Case 5: Watershed cerebral infarction

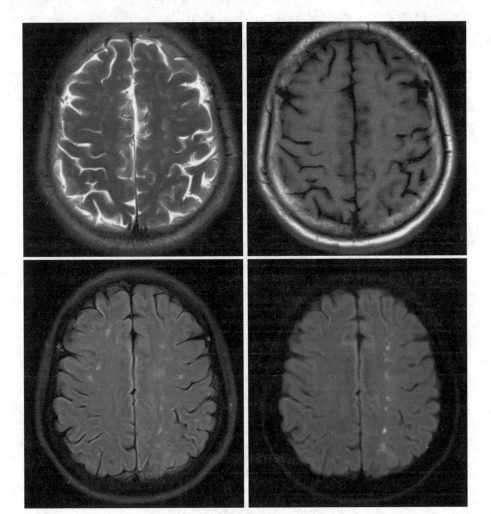

图 3-1-5 分水岭脑梗死

Findings

No abnormality was observed in scalp soft tissue and skull bone structure. Several small speckled and patchlike T2WI and FLAIR slightly high signal shadow were observed in bilateral frontal and parietal lobes, lateral ventricles, and central white matter area of semi-ovale. T1WI was not clear, and the boundary was basically clear. Multiple patchy and speckled high signals can be seen in the left frontal parietal lobe, semioval center, and near the posterior horn of the left ventricle in the DWI sequence, and the display is relatively clear.The ventricles, sulcus and cistern were slightly widened and deepened. Symmetrical patchiness of slightly longer T1 and slightly longer T2 signal shadows could be seen near the anterior and posterior horns of bilateral ventricles. FLAIR sequence showed high signal.No space-occupying lesions were observed in the sellar region and bilateral cerebellar pontine Angle. The midline structure is centered. Bilateral ethmoid sinuses and bilateral inferior turbinate mucosa were thickened.

Impression

(1) Mixed watershed cerebral infarction on the left.

(2) Ischemic white matter lesions (Fazekas Ⅱ grade).

(3) Bilateral ethmoid sinusitis, double inferior turbinate hypertrophy.

病例5：分水岭脑梗死

征象描述

头皮软组织及颅骨骨质结构未见异常。于双额顶叶、侧脑室体旁、半卵圆中心白质区见多个小斑点状及斑片状T2WI与FLAIR稍高信号影，T1WI显示不明确，边界基本清晰。DWI序列左额顶叶、半卵圆中心、左侧脑室后角旁可见多发斑斑片状及斑点状高信号，显示较清晰。脑室、脑沟、脑池稍增宽加深，双侧脑室前后角旁可见对称性斑片状稍长T1稍长T2信号影，FLAIR序列呈高信号。鞍区及双侧脑桥小脑角区未见占位性病变。中线结构居中。双侧筛窦及双下鼻甲黏膜增厚。

影像诊断

(1) 左侧混合型分水岭脑梗死。

(2) 缺血性脑白质病变（Fazekas Ⅱ级）。

(3) 双侧筛窦炎、双下鼻甲肥大。

Case 6: Intracerebral hemorrhage in the left external capsule area (subacute stage)

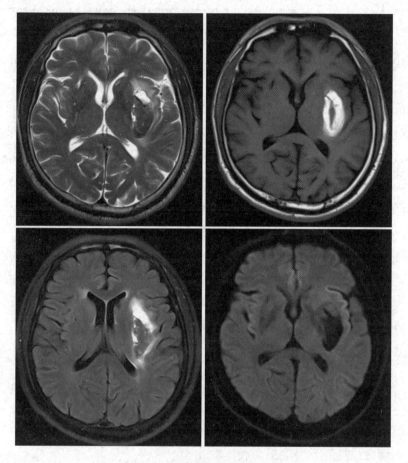

图 3-1-6　左侧外囊区亚急性期脑出血

Findings

No abnormality was observed in scalp soft tissue and skull bone structure. An elliptical abnormal signal shadow was observed in the left external capsule area. T1WI showed central low signal change and edge high signal change, and T2WI and FLAIR showed high and low mixed signal change, DWI sequence showed low signal change, the size was about 23mm×31mm×44mm, patchlike slightly longer T1 and slightly longer T2 signal shadow around the focal area, and the adjacent sulcus was compressed and narrowed. Multiple small round long T1 and long T2 signal shadows can be seen in the right basal ganglia region and corona radiata, and FLAIR sequences show low signal shadows in the center and high signal shadows in the edge. Multiple speckled T2WI and FLAIR slightly high signal shadows were seen in the white matter area of bilateral frontal lobes, corona radiata and center of semiovale. The T1WI display was not clear and the boundary was not clear.The ventricles, sulcus and cistern were clearly displayed. Symmetrical patchiness of slightly longer T1 and slightly longer T2 signals could be seen near the anterior and posterior horns of bilateral ventricles. FLAIR sequence showed high signal.No space-occupying lesions were observed in the sellar region and bilateral cerebellar pontine Angle. The midline structure is centered. The mucosa of the ethmoid sinuses is thickened on both sides, and the double inferior turbinate is thickened.

Impression

(1) Intracerebral hemorrhage in the left external capsule area (subacute stage) with perifocal edema and superior thalamic infarction.

(2) Multiple old lacunar cerebral infarction in the right basal ganglia region and corona radiata.

(3) Ischemic white matter lesions (Fazekas Ⅰ grade).

病例6：左侧外囊区亚急性期脑出血

征象描述

头皮软组织及颅骨骨质结构未见异常。于左侧外囊区见一类椭圆形异常信号影，T1WI呈中央低信号边缘高信号改变，T2WI及FLAIR呈高低混杂信号改变，DWI序列呈低信号，大小约为23mm×31mm×44mm，灶周可见斑片状稍长T1稍长T2信号影环绕，邻近脑沟裂受压变窄。右侧基底节区及放射冠可见多发小类圆形长T1长T2信号影，FLAIR序列呈中央低信号边缘高信号影。双额叶白质区、放射冠、半卵圆中心见多个小斑点状T2WI与FLAIR稍高信号影，T1WI显示不明确，边界欠清。脑室、脑沟、脑池显示清晰，双侧脑室前后角旁可见对称性斑片状稍长T1稍长

T2 信号影，FLAIR 序列呈高信号。鞍区及双侧脑桥小脑角区未见占位性病变。中线结构居中。双侧筛窦黏膜增厚，双下鼻甲肥厚。

影像诊断

(1) 左侧外囊区脑出血（亚急性期）伴灶周水肿、上丘脑梗死。

(2) 右侧基底节区及放射冠多发陈旧性腔隙性脑梗死。

(3) 缺血性脑白质病变（Fazekas Ⅰ级）。

Case 7: Acute pancreatitis

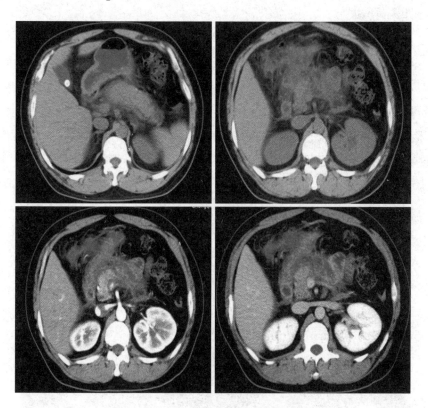

图 3-1-7　急性胰腺炎合并胆囊结石

Findings

The pancreas is enlarged in volume, with full contour, blurred boundary, low parenchyma density. CT value of 37HU, lower density area can be seen in the body of pancreas, CT value of 21HU, the pancreatic duct is not significantly dilated. Fat space between pancreas, stomach and small intestine is blurred, obvious peripancreatic exudate can be seen. Left anterior renal fascia is thickened, interintestinal and lesser omental sac can be seen exudate. Enhanced scanning of the pancreatic body and tail showed poor enhancement, enlarged gallbladder, and smooth cyst wall and no obvious thickening, with high-density stone shadows inside. No obvious dilatation of intrahepatic and extrahepatic bile ducts was observed.

Impression

(1) Acute pancreatitis with peripancreatic exudation and possible partial necrosis.

(2) Gallbladder stones.

病例7：急性胰腺炎

征象描述

胰腺体积增大，轮廓饱满，边界模糊，实质密度较低，CT值37Hu，胰体部内可见更低密度区，CT值21Hu，胰管未见明显扩张，胰腺与胃、小肠间脂肪间隙模糊，胰周见明显渗出液，左侧肾前筋膜增厚，肠间、小网膜囊内可见渗液，增强扫描胰体尾强化稍差，胆囊增大，囊壁尚光整，未见明显增厚，其内见高密度结石影；肝内外胆管未见明显扩张。

影像诊断

(1) 急性胰腺炎伴胰周渗出，部分坏死可能。

(2) 胆囊结石。

Case 8: Epidural hematoma

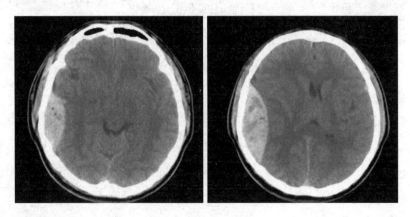

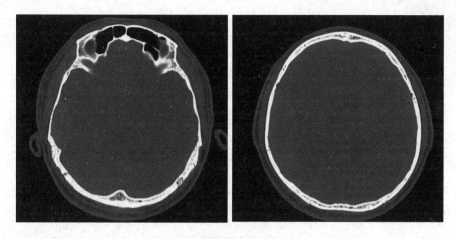

图 3-1-8 右颞顶部硬膜外血肿

Findings

A biconvex high-density shadow was observed under the right temporal cranial plate, with a size of about 77mm×26mm, showing mass effect. The right lateral ventricle was compressed and the midline structure of the brain shifts to the left. Multiple linear low-density shadows were observed in the right temporal bone with bone interruption, and fluid density shadows were observed in the right mastoid air chamber and external auditory canal. Patchy high-density shadow was seen below the left temporal cranial plate, and slightly low-density shadow was seen around the focal area.Bilateral temporal swelling of the soft tissues can be seen. Thickening of mucosa was seen in bilateral ethmoid sinus and right sphenoid sinus.

Impression

(1) Right temporal bone and parietal bone fracture accompanied by right epidural hematoma and left parietal lobe offset brain contusion. Short-term reexamination is recommended.

(2) Fracture of mastoid process of right temporal bone with effusion of air chamber in mastoid process.Bilateral temporal soft tissue swelling

病例 8：右颞顶部硬膜外血肿

征象描述

右侧颞部颅板下见双凸形高密度影，大小约 77mm×26mm，可见占位效应，右侧侧脑室受压、脑中线结构左移；右侧颞骨骨质中断，见多发线状低密度影，右侧乳突气房、外耳道见液体密度影。左侧颞部颅板下见条片状高密度影，灶周见稍低密度影环绕。双侧颞部软组织肿胀。双侧筛窦、右侧蝶窦见黏膜增厚影。

影像诊断

(1) 右侧颞骨、顶骨骨折并右侧硬膜外血肿、左顶叶对冲性脑挫伤，建议短期复查。

(2) 右侧颞骨乳突部骨折并右侧乳突气房积液，双侧颞部软组织肿胀。

Case 9: Colles fracture of right distal radius

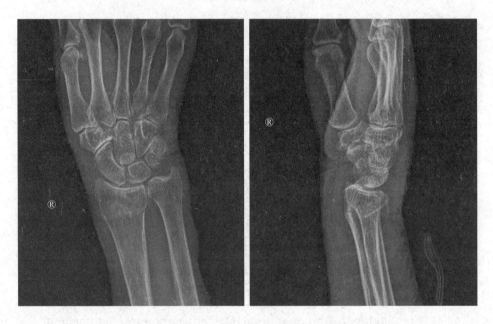

图 3-1-9　右桡骨远端骨折

Findings

Bone fracture of the distal radius on the right side shows a clear fracture line shadow. The broken end shifts to the dorsal side, and the surrounding soft tissue is swollen. No obvious signs of fracture and dislocation were observed in the remaining bones, and the joint space was clear.

Impression

Colles fracture of right distal radius.

病例 9：右桡骨远端骨折

征象描述

右侧侧桡骨远端骨质断裂，见透亮骨折线影，断端向背侧移位，周围软组织肿胀。余诸骨未见明显骨折及脱位征象，所见关节间隙清晰。

影像诊断

右侧桡骨远端 colles 骨折。

Case 10: Aseptic necrosis of the femoral head on both sides

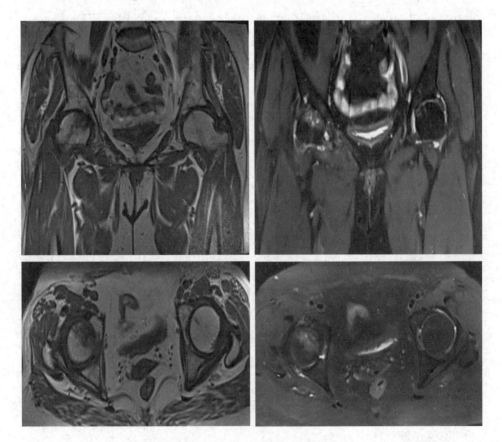

图 3-1-10　两侧股骨头无菌性坏死

Description of image

The hip joint space on the right side was slightly narrowed and the articular surface was rough. The articular surface of the right femoral head was slightly collapsed, and most of the articular cartilage structure disappeared. Multiple patchy long T1 and long T2 signal shadows could be seen under the articular surface and in the femoral neck, with blurred edges. Multiple small cystic and patchlike long T1 and T2 signal shadows were observed in bilateral acetabulum. There was no narrowing of the left joint space, patchy long T1 and long T2 signal shadows were seen under the articular surface of the femoral head, with blurred edges, and no obvious collapse of the articular surface. Small cystic long T1 and long T2 signal shadows were also seen in the posterior part of the iliac wings on both sides, with clear margins. No abnormal changes were observed in bilateral sacroiliac joints.

Impression

(1) Aseptic necrosis of the femoral head on both sides (stage Ⅲ on the right side, stage Ⅱ on the left).

(2) Multiple cystic lesions in bilateral acetabulum and posterior iliac wing.

病例 10：两侧股骨头无菌性坏死

征象描述

右侧髋关节间隙稍变窄，关节面毛糙。右侧股骨头关节面稍塌陷，关节面软骨结构大部分消失，关节面下及股骨颈可见多发斑片状长 T1 长 T2 信号影，边缘模糊。双侧髋臼可见多发小囊状及斑片状长 T1 长 T2 信号影。左侧关节间隙未见变窄，股骨头关节面下可见斑片状长 T1 长 T2 信号影，边缘模糊，关节面未见明显塌陷。两侧髂骨翼后部也可见小囊状长 T1 长 T2 信号影，边缘清楚。两侧骶髂关节未见异常改变。

影像诊断

(1) 两侧股骨头无菌性坏死（右侧Ⅲ期、左侧Ⅱ期）。

(2) 双侧髋臼及髂骨翼后部多发囊变灶。

Case 11: Osteofibrous dysplasia in the right temporal bone

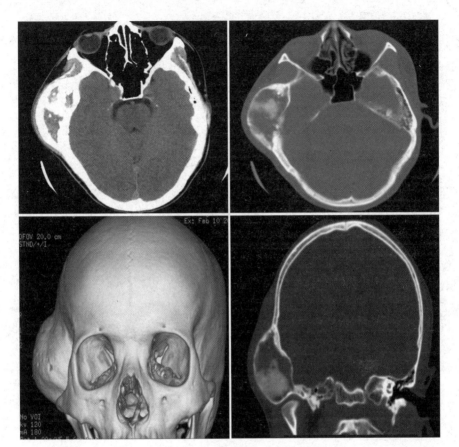

图 3-1-11 颞骨骨纤维结构不良

Findings

There was a large irregular bony bulge on the right side of the temporal bone, with uneven internal density, as well as high-density clumpy, dotted and soft tissue density shadow. The soft tissue density CT value was 40HU, and the size was about 4.0×6.2cm. The peripheral bony margin had different degrees of bone absorption, but the margin was still clear. No obvious abnormal density shadow was observed in each intracranial part. No obvious abnormalities were observed in the ventricle system, sulci and cistern. The midline structure has no shift. Multiple soft tissue shadows in the left maxillary sinus were scanned horizontally.

Impression

(1) The right temporal bone changes, considering benign bone tumors or tumor-like lesions, the possibility of osteofibrous dysplasia is high.

(2) Inflammation of the left maxillary sinus.

病例11：右颞骨骨纤维结构不良

征象描述

右侧颞骨见一较大不规则骨性隆起块影，其内密度不均，并可见高密度团状、点状及软组织密度影，软组织密度CT值40HU，大小约4.0cm×6.2cm，周围骨性边缘不同程度骨质吸收，但边缘尚清楚，大脑、小脑及脑干形态、大小未见明显异常，颅内各部未见明显异常密度影；脑室系统、脑沟以及脑池未见明显异常；中线结构无移位；扫描水平左侧上颌窦增多软组织影。

影像诊断

(1) 右侧颞骨改变，考虑良性骨肿瘤性或肿瘤样病变，骨纤维结构不良可能性大。

(2) 左侧上颌窦炎症。

Case 12: Left kidney cancer

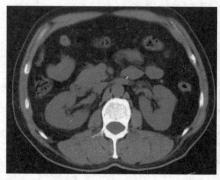
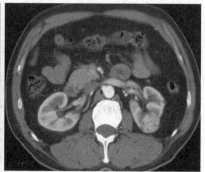

图 3-1-12　左肾癌

Findings

The shape and size of the liver were normal. A small round cystic low-density shadow was observed in the left outer lobe of the liver. No enhancement was observed after enhancement.

No abnormal density shadow was observed in the remaining liver parenchyma, and no obvious abnormal enhancement was observed after enhancement scanning. The gallbladder is not large, the wall is not obvious thickened, and there is no abnormal density shadow in the cyst cavity. No dilatation of intrahepatic bile duct was observed. The shape and size of the spleen were normal, and the parenchymal density was uniform. No abnormal enhancement was observed after enhancement. No abnormality was observed in the shape and size of the pancreas. The parenchyma was uniform in density and the peripancreatic fat space was clear. The size was about 2.5cm×3.0cm. The plain scan CT value was about 39HU, and showed uneven after enhancement. The CT values of arterial phase, venous phase and delayed phase were about 96-157HU, 94-116HU, and 85-93HU, respectively. The perirenal space is clear. There was no obvious abnormality in the shape, size and density of bilateral adrenal glands. No obvious enlargement of lymph nodes was observed retroperitoneal. No effusion was observed in the abdominal cavity.

Impression

(1) Circular space occupation in left renal parenchyma, neoplastic lesions and renal cancer are considered. High chance of renal cancer and further examination is recommended.

(2) Multiple cysts in both kidneys.

(3) Small cyst of left outer lobe of liver.

(4) A few fibrous strip foci in the bottom of both lungs.

病例12：左肾癌

征象描述

肝脏形态、大小正常，肝左外叶见小类圆形囊性低密度影，增强后无强化，余肝实质内未见异常密度影，增强扫描后未见明显异常强化影。胆囊不大，壁未见明显增厚，囊腔内未见异常密度影；肝内胆管未见扩张。

脾脏形态、大小正常，实质密度均匀，增强后未见明显异常强化灶。胰腺形态、大小未见异常，实质密度均匀，胰周脂肪间隙清晰。左肾实质内见类圆形等密度占位，边界较清楚，大小约 2.5cm×3.0cm，平扫 CT 值约 39HU，增强后呈不均匀强化，动脉期、静脉期、延迟期 CT 值分别约为 96-157HU、94-116HU、85-93HU，双肾多发囊性无强化低密度椭圆形影，双肾周间隙清晰。双侧肾上腺形态、大小及密度未见明显异常。腹膜后未见明显肿大淋巴结影。腹腔未见积液。

影像诊断

(1) 左肾实质内类圆形占位，考虑肿瘤性病变，肾癌可能性大，建议进一步检查。

(2) 双肾多发囊肿。

(3) 肝左外叶小囊肿。

(4) 双肺底少许纤维条索灶。

第二章　医学影像诊断报告

一、医学 X 线平片诊断报告（Medical X-Ray reports）

X-Ray Report 1

Technique

Hands and wrists, two views

Findings

Hands and wrists, two views of the right and left hand and wrist were obtained. There is generalized osteopenia. There are OA changes seen at the first CMC joint with subchondral sclerosis and joint space narrowing. Ulnar styloids appear intact. There is no chondrocalcinosis. There are some degenerative changes seen at the carpus but without any obvious erosive changes. There are no erosions seen at any of the MCP or PIP joints. There are scattered areas of joint space narrowing at the PIP and DIP joints.

Impression

(1) Osteoarthritis changes.

(2) Osteopenia.

(3) No definite erosions.

X-Ray Report 2

Technique

Chest, two views.

第三部分 医学影像诊断病例及影像报告

Findings

The lungs are well aerated. There is no evidence of any focal area of consolidation. A faint rounded density is seen in the base of the left lower hemithorax probably representing a nipple shadow. The hilar and pulmonary vasculature is normal. The heart size is within normal limits. The costophrenic angles are clear.

Impression

Normal chest X-ray.

X-Ray Report 3

Technique

Left foot, sagittal, axial and coronal views.

Findings

Three view of the left foot show no evidence of fracture, dislocation, or other acute bony abnormality.

Impression

Negative left foot films.

X-Ray Report 4

Technique

Right shoulder, two views

Findings

Lumbosacral spine, multiple views of the lumbar spine were obtained. There appears to be a fracture at the coccyx which is age indeterminate. There is straightening of normal lumbar lordosis. Intervertebral disc spaces are maintained. Facet joints appear within normal limits bilaterally. There is a little bit of sacroiliac sclerosis bilaterally, more so on the right. The SI joints do appear patent.

Impression

(1) Suspected coccyx fracture, age indeterminate.

(2) Straightening of the lumbar lordosis.

(3) Sacroiliac sclerosis.

X-Ray Report 5

Technique

Hips, two views.

Findings

Hips, two views of the right and left hip were obtained. Bony mineralization is normal. There is no acute fracture seen. There is no visible enthesopathy in the limited views of the pelvis. There is a little bit of superior sclerosis at the acetabula bilaterally. The hip joint spaces appear preserved.

Impression

(1) Mild hip sclerosis.

(2) Otherwise, unremarkable hips.

X-Ray Report 6

Technique

Lumbar spine, two views.

Findings

No fractures, subluxations or other acute bony abnormalities are identified. There is mild degenerative change with mild endplate spur formation and mild facet sclerosis at all levels. No erosive or destructive changes are seen.

Impression

(1) Mild degenerative changes as described above.

(2) No definite acute abnormality.

二、医学CT诊断报告（Medical CT reports）

CT Abdomen Report 1

CT of the upper abdomen with contrast.

Clinical history

Follow-up aneurysms.

Technique

CT was performed of the upper abdomen following the administration of IV contrast utilizing standard protocol. The current study is compared to a prior CT examination of the abdomen from 03/08/05 and a prior MRI of the upper abdomen from 09/07/05.

Findings

No focal liver lesions are identified. There is mild dilatation of the common bowel duct and intrahepatic biliary radicals. This was present on the previous study. It appears unchanged. There is no evidence of splenic enlargement. The spleen is imaged in the splenic arterial phase and is therefore inhomogeneous.

The adrenals are not enlarged. No intrarenal mass is identified.

There was no visible pancreatic mass. There was no evidence of dilatation of the small bowel or colon.

Maximum transverse diameter of the large fusiform aneurysm of the infrarenal aorta is now 7.8 cm. This demonstrates continued growth when compared to the prior MRI. There is a very large mural thrombus noted in association with this aneurysm.

The aneurysm at the level of the aortic hiatus is described on the CT chest report. This aneurysm also contains a large amount of mural thrombus.

There was no evidence of ascites or free fluid within the abdomen. There was no evidence of retroperitoneal hemorrhage at this time.

Impression

The infrarenal aneurysm of the abdominal aorta has increased in size as described above.

CT Left Shoulder Report 2

Noncontrast CT of the left shoulder.

Clinical history

Left shoulder pain.

Technique

Standard noncontrast shoulder technique.

Findings

The obvious structures are intact. There is no dislocation. The infraspinatus and teres minor tendons are maintained. There is a focal vertical tear of the supraspinatus tendon at the insertion, which appears full thickness. There is no tendon retraction. The subscapularis tendon is intact.

The long head of the biceps tendon is in anatomic location and the biceps anchor is maintained. There is no detached labral tear.

The acromioclavicular joint is unremarkable. There is no glenohumeral joint effusion. There is no disproportionate muscle atrophy.

Impression

Focal vertical/linear full-thickness tear of the supraspinatus tendon laterally at the insertion. No evidence for tendon retraction.

CT Lumbar Spine Report 3

CT of the lumbar spine.

Clinical history

Low back pain radiating into both legs.

Technique

CT was performed of the lumbar spine utilizing standard protocol.

Sagittal and coronal reconstructions were utilized for this examination. The current study is compared to an MRI of the lumbar spine performed the same day.

Findings

There are five vertebrae with lumbar configuration. There is a 4.5 cm×2.7 cm cystic structure noted on the lowest cut of the examination to the right of midline. This may represent a right adnexal cyst. Correlation with pelvic sonography is recommended.

There is preservation of the normal lumbar lordosis. There is 4-mm retrolisthesis of L2 on L3. 4-mm retrolisthesis of L3 on L4 and 2-mm retrolisthesis of L4 on L5. There is subchondral sclerosis involving the inferior endplates of L2, L3 and L4 and superior endplates of L3 and L4.

There is calcification of the annulus at the L5-S1 level.

At the T12-L1 and L1-L2 levels, no significant abnormality is detected.

At the L2-L3 level, there is moderate loss of height of the disc. There is retrolisthesis of L2 on L3 as described above. A diffuse annular bulge is present. The central canal is diminished in cross-sectional area without evidence of central spinal stenosis. There is no evidence of significant facet spurring or foraminal narrowing.

At the L3-L4 level, there is severe loss of height of the disc. As noted above, there is a prominent retrolisthesis of L3 on L4. There is a mild diffuse annular bulge present. The central canal appears adequate in caliber. There is evidence of bilateral facet hypertrophy with mild foraminal narrowing on the left.

At the L4-L5 level, there is severe loss of height of the disc and a mild retrolisthesis of L4 on L5. A mild diffuse annular bulge is present. There is a droplet of nitrogen gas in the left anterior epidural space indicating the presence of a radial tear of the annulus. However, there is no evidence of focal disc protrusion. The central canal appears adequate in caliber. There is bilateral facet hypertrophy with calcification of the joint capsules bilaterally. There is mild foraminal narrowing on the left.

At the L5-S1 level, disc height is preserved. The posterior margin of the disc appears unremarkable. The central canal is adequate in caliber. There is evidence of bilateral facet spurring without significant foraminal narrowing

Impression

Diffuse degenerative changes without evidence of focal disc protrusion as described above. The changes are similar to those noted on the MRI. Please see complete discussion above.

CT Sinuses Report 4

CT sinuses without contrast.

Clinical history

Sinus infection.

Technique

Noncontrast CT of the paranasal sinuses was performed.

Findings

There is slight rightward deviation of the anterior aspect of the nasal septum. The nasal turbinates are within normal limits. There is normal aeration of the paranasal sinuses, without mucosal thickening or opacification. There is no air-fluid level identified. The ostiomeatal units appear patent.

The facial and orbital soft tissue structures are within normal limits. There is no fluid collection or inflammatory stranding.

Impression

Within normal limits. No sinus inflammatory changes identified.

三、MRI 诊断报告 (Medical MRI reports)

MRI Brain Report 1

Technique

MRI was performed of the brain prior to and following the administration of IV gadolinium utilizing standard protocol. No prior study is available for comparison.

Findings

The basilar cisterns, ventricular system and cortical sulci appear unremarkable for a 67-year-old patient. The visualized mastoid air cells and paranasal sinuses appear clear. There are multiple small foci of increased signal on T2 weighted and FLAIR images in the subcortical white matter, predominately in the frontal regions of both hemispheres. There is no evidence of mass effect, midline shift, extra-axial fluid collection or hemorrhage. There are no abnormal areas of contrast enhancement identified within the brain.

The pituitary is not enlarged. The cerebellar tonsils are in normal anatomic position. The Ⅶ-Ⅷ nerve complexes have a symmetric and unremarkable appearance without evidence of abnormal contrast enhancement.

Impression

Focal abnormalities in the white matter as described above are generally associated with ischemic microvascular disease. A demyelinating process can have a similar appearance. Clinical correlation is suggested. See complete discussion above.

MRI Brain Report 2

Technique

MRI examination of the brain is performed using the following protocol: T1 weighted sagittal and coronal, T2 weighted coronal, FLAIR and T1 weighted axial sequences. The patient refused contrast enhancement so post-contrast scans have not been done. Also, please note that diffusion scans have not been done.

Findings

The brain parenchyma shows normal signal intensity on the various pulse sequences. There is no intracranial mass, mass effect or area of abnormal signal intensity. The right temporal horn is slightly prominent and asymmetric. Flow voids are appreciated in the major intracranial vessels.

Impression

Normal noncontrast mai examination of the brain. Please note that diffusion-weighted scans have not been done.

MRI Brain IAC Report 3

Technique

MRI of the brain was performed using a combination of T1 and T2 weighted axial, sagittal and coronal images. Additional thin section images were also obtained through the cerebellopontine angles for evaluation of the internal auditory canals.

Findings

The brain parenchyma shows normal signal intensity. There is no confluent edema or mass effect. There is no extra-axial collection identified. The corpus callosum is well formed and it is in good position. The cerebellar tonsils are unremarkable. The pituitary gland is normal in size. The cavernous sinuses are symmetric. The basal cisterns are symmetric in appearance.

The cerebellopontine angle cisterns are normal in appearance, without mass or mass effect. The VII and VIII nerve complexes are unremarkable. There is no evidence for vestibular schwannoma or other mass. Trigeminal nerves are symmetric in caliber and in normal position. There are normal flow voids in the basilar artery and along the circle of Willis.

Impression

The exam is within normal limits. The brain parenchyma is normal in appearance, without edema or mass identified. Cerebellopontine angle cisterns are intact, without evidence for vestibular schwannoma or other abnormality.

MRI Knee Report 4

Technique

Multiple pulsing sequences are performed at three planes with emphasis on T1, proton density, and T2 weighting.

Findings

There are moderate intrameniscal myxoid changes in the medial meniscus. The intrameniscal myxoid changes are more pronounced in the posterior horn. There is no evidence of discrete meniscal tear extending to an articular surface in a linear fashion of either the medial or lateral meniscus. The anterior and posterior cruciate ligaments are intact. There is some edema medial to the MCL consistent with a grade I MCL sprain. There is also some fluid deep to the MCL below the joint line consistent with some TCL bursitis. There is a fairly large broad band of edema in the medial tibial plateau extending to the medial aspect of the lateral tibial plateau compatible with an area of edema, or contusion. There is some subchondral degenerative changes in the femoral condyle. A discrete fracture line is not identified. The lateral collateral ligament appears intact. The extensor mechanism appears intact. There is chondromalacia patella most pronounced along the lateral facet as well as the lateral aspect of the medial facet near the patellar apex. The chondromalacia patella is most pronounced at the level of the upper pole of the patella. A few small subchondral cysts are seen within the patella. There is a small joint effusion.

Impression

(1) Grade I MCL sprain.

(2) TCL bursitis.

(3) Band of edema or contusion throughout the medial aspect of the proximal tibia as noted above.

(4) Medial compartment degenerative changes with intrameniscal myxoid changes within the medial meniscus. No evidence of franc Meniscal tear.

(5) Small joint effusion.

(6) Chondromalacia patella.

MRI Lumbar Spine Report 5

Clinical history

Low back pain, radiating to both thighs.

Technique

MRI examination of the lumbar spine is performed using the following protocol: T1 weighted and T2 weighted axial and sagittal sequences.

Findings

The lumbar vertebral alignment is well maintained. The vertebral body heights and disc spaces are well maintained. Normal T2 hyperintensities are seen within all the discs in the lumbar spine. Axial scans are done from disc space level L2-L3 through L5-S1. At disc space levels L4-L5 and L5-S1, there are very minimal diffuse disc bulges. There is no focal disc herniation, canal stenosis or foraminal narrowing seen at any of the levels in the lumbar spine.

Impression

(1) Very minimal diffuse disc bulges seen at levels L4-L5 and L5-S1.

(2) There is no disc herniation, canal stenosis or foraminal narrowing seen at any of the levels in the lumbar spine.

MRI Right Shoulder Report 6

Clinical history

Impingement.

Technique

Use the standard noncontrast technique.

Findings

The infraspinatus and teres minor tendons are intact. There is mild tendinosis of the supraspinatus tendon without tear. The subscapularis tendon is intact. The long head of the biceps tendon is in anatomic location and the biceps anchor is maintained.

There is moderate degenerative arthrosis of the AC joint and slight thickening of the coracoacromial ligament. These may contribute to clinical impingement. There is no joint effusion or disproportionate muscle atrophy.

Impression

(1) Mild tendinosis of the supraspinatus tendon without tear.

(2) Moderate DJD of the AC joint with slight thickening or the coracoacromial ligament. These may contribute to clinical impingement.

四、超声诊断报告（Diagnostic Ultrasound Reports）

Gallbladder Ultrasound Report 1

Examination

Gallbladder ultrasound.

Findings

The gallbladder appears normal. There is no gallstones, gallbladder wall thickening or pericholecystic fluid. There is no notation of the intra or extrahepatic biliary system. The common bile duct measures 1.1 cm

Impression

No sonographic abnormality of the gallbladder is identified.

Renal Ultrasound Report 2

Examination

Renal ultrasound.

Findings

The right kidney measures 9 cm in length and the left kidney measures approximately 10.6 cm in length. There is no hydronephrosis, nephrolithiasis or renal mass. There is no perinephric fluid collection.

Impression

No sonographic abnormality of the kidneys is identified.

Scrotal Ultrasound Report 3

Examination

Scrotal ultrasound.

Findings

Both testicles are normal in size, contour and echogenicity. The right testicle measures 5.2 cm×2.2 cm×3.6 cm and the left testicle measures 5.0 cm×2.3 cm×3.3 cm. There is normal Doppler flow to both testicles. The right epididymis measures 1.0 cm×0.3 cm×0.3 cm. The left epididymis is slightly larger measuring 1.1 cm×0.7 cm×0.5 cm.

There is a normal amount of fluid within the scrotum. There is no hernia identified within the right groin containing bowel.

Impression

Negative scrotal ultrasound.

Venous Doppler Report 4

Examination

Bilateral lower extremity venous doppler.

Findings

Both common femoral veins, superficial femoral veins, popliteal veins and posterior tibial veins exhibited normal flow, compressibility and augmentation.

Impression

No evidence of deep venous thrombosis in either leg.

Shoulder Ultrasound Report 5

Examination

Ultrasound of the Shoulder.

Clinical History

Shoulder pain, evaluate for rotator cuff abnormality.

Findings

No evidence of joint effusion. The biceps brachii long head tendon is normal without tendinosis, tear, tenosynovitis, or subluxation/dislocation. The supraspinatus, infraspinatus, subscapularis, and teres minor tendons are also normal. No subacromial-subdeltoid bursal abnormality and no sonographic evidence for subacromial impingement with dynamic maneuvers. The posterior labrum is unremarkable. Additional focused evaluation at site of maximal symptoms was unrevealing.

Impression

Unremarkable ultrasound examination of the shoulder. No rotator cuff abnormality.

Shoulder Ultrasound Report 6

Examination

Ultrasound of the Shoulder.

Clinical History

Shoulder pain, evaluate for rotator cuff abnormality.

Findings

There is a focal anechoic tear of the anterior, distal aspect of the supraspinatus tendon measuring 1 cm short axis by 1.5 cm long axis. The anterior margin of the tear is adjacent to the rotator interval. There is no involvement of the subscapularis, infraspinatus, or rotator interval. A moderate amount of infraspinatus and supraspinatus fatty degeneration is present. There is a small joint effusion distending the biceps brachii tendon sheath and moderate distention of the subacromial-subdeltoid bursa. No biceps brachii long head tendon abnormality and no subluxation/dislocation. Mild osteoarthritis of the acromioclavicular joint. Additional focused evaluation at site of maximal symptoms was unrevealing.

Impression

Focal or incomplete full-thickness tear of the supraspinatus tendon with infraspinatus and supraspinatus muscle atrophy.

Elbow Ultrasound Report 7

Examination

Ultrasound of the Elbow.

Clinical History

Elbow pain, evaluate for tendon abnormality.

Findings

No evidence of joint effusion or synovial process. The biceps brachii and brachialis are normal. The common flexor and extensor tendons are also normal. No significant triceps brachii abnormality. The anterior bundle of the ulnar collateral ligament and lateral collateral ligament complex are normal. The ulnar nerve, radial nerve, and median nerve at the elbow are unremarkable. No abnormality in the cubital tunnel region with dynamic imaging. Additional focused evaluation at site of maximal symptoms was unrevealing.

Impression

Unremarkable ultrasound examination of the elbow.

Elbow Ultrasound Report 8

Examination

Ultrasound of the Elbow.

Clinical History

Elbow pain, evaluate for tendon abnormality.

Findings

There is a partial-thickness tear of the distal biceps brachii tendon involving the superficial short head tendon with approximately 2 cm of retraction but with intact long head. Dynamic evaluation shows continuity of the long head excluding full-thickness tear. No joint effusion. The triceps brachii, common extensor, and common flexor tendons are normal. The ulnar, radial, and median nerves are unremarkable, including dynamic evaluation of the ulnar nerve. Unremarkable ulnar and lateral collateral ligaments. No bursal distention.

Impression

Partial-thickness tear of the distal biceps brachii tendon.

Wrist Ultrasound Report 9

Examination

Ultrasound of the Wrist.

Clinical History

Numbness, evaluate for carpal tunnel syndrome.

Findings

The median nerve is unremarkable in appearance, measuring 8mm 2 at the wrist crease and 7mm 2 at the pronator quadratus. No evidence of tenosynovitis. The radiocarpal, midcarpal, and distal radioulnar joints are normal without effusion or synovial hypertrophy. The wrist tendons are normal without tear or tenosynovitis. Normal dorsal component of the scapholunate ligament. No dorsal or volar ganglion cyst. Unremarkable Guyon canal. Additional focused evaluation at site of maximal symptoms was unrevealing.

Impression

Unremarkable ultrasound examination of the wrist.

Diagnostic Wrist Ultrasound Report 10

Examination

Ultrasound of the Wrist.

Clinical History

Numbness, evaluate for carpal tunnel syndrome

Findings

The median nerve is hypoechoic and enlarged, measuring 15mm at the wrist crease and 7mm at the pronator quadratus. No evidence for tenosynovitis. The radiocarpal, midcarpal, and distal radioulnar joints are normal without effusion or synovial hypertrophy. The wrist tendons are normal without tear or tenosynovitis. Normal dorsal component of the scapholunate ligament. No dorsal ganglion cyst. A 7-mm volar ganglion cyst is noted between the radial artery and flexor carpi radialis tendon. Unremarkable Guyon canal. Additional focused evaluation at site of maximal symptoms was unrevealing.

Impression

(1) Ultrasound findings compatible with carpal tunnel syndrome.

(2) A 7-mm volar ganglion cyst.

Hip Ultrasound Report 11

Examination

Ultrasound of the Right Hip.

Clinical History

Hip pain, evaluate for bursitis.

Findings

The hip joint is normal without effusion or synovial hypertrophy.

Limited evaluation of the anterior labrum is unremarkable. No evidence of iliopsoas bursal distention or snapping iliopsoas tendon with dynamic imaging. The remaining anterior tendons, including the rectus femoris and sartorius, as well as the adductors, are normal. Evaluation of the lateral hip is normal. No evidence of abnormal bursal distention around the greater trochanter. The gluteus minimus and medius tendons are normal. No abnormal snapping with dynamic evaluation.

Impression

Unremarkable ultrasound examination of the hip.

Hip Ultrasound Report 12

Examination

Ultrasound of the Right Hip.

Clinical History

Hip pain, evaluate for tendon tear.

Findings

There is a partial tear of the adductor longus origin at the pubis. No evidence of full-thickness tear or tendon retraction. The common aponeurosis and rectus abdominis tendon are normal, as is the pubic symphysis. The hip joint is normal without effusion or synovial hypertrophy. There is a possible tear of the anterior labrum. No paralabral cyst. No evidence of iliopsoas bursal distention or snapping iliopsoas tendon with dynamic imaging. Evaluation of the lateral hip is normal. No evidence of abnormal bursal distention around the greater trochanter. The gluteus minimus and medius tendons are normal. No abnormal snapping with dynamic evaluation.

Impression

(1) Partial-thickness tear of the proximal adductor longus.

(2) Possible anterior labral tear. Consider MR arthrography if indicated.

Knee Ultrasound Report 13

Examination

Ultrasound of the Right Knee.

Clinical History

Trauma.

Findings

The extensor mechanism, including the quadriceps tendon, patella, and patellar tendon, is normal without bursal abnormalities. No significant joint effusion or synovial hypertrophy. The medial collateral and lateral collateral ligaments are normal. Unremarkable iliotibial tract, biceps femoris, popliteus tendon, and common peroneal nerve. No Baker cyst. Limited evaluation of the menisci is unremarkable.

Impression

Unremarkable ultrasound examination of the right knee.

Knee Ultrasound Report 14

Examination

Ultrasound of the Right Knee.

Clinical History

Pain, evaluate for cyst.

Findings

The extensor mechanism, including the quadriceps tendon, patella, and patellar tendon, is normal. There is a moderate-sized joint effusion and no synovial hypertrophy or intra-articular body. The medial and lateral collateral ligaments are normal, as is the iliotibial tract, biceps femoris, popliteus tendon, and common peroneal nerve. There is medial compartment joint space narrowing and osteophyte formation with mild extrusion of the body of the medial meniscus, which is abnormally hypoechoic. No parameniscal cyst. There is a Baker cyst measuring 2 cm× 2 cm× 6 cm. Abnormal hypoechogenicity is noted at the inferior margin of the Baker cyst. There is also a hypoechoic cleft involving the posterior horn of the medial meniscus, which extends to the articular surface.

Impression

(1) Baker cyst with evidence for rupture.

(2) Medial compartment osteoarthritis with moderate joint effusion.

(3) Suspect posterior horn medial meniscal tear. Consider MRI for confirmation if indicated.

附录　国外影像医学临床与教学

第一章　美国医学影像学教育与培训
（Education and Training of Medical Imaging in the United States）

在美国，要成为一个真正的放射（影像）科医师，必须经历一个非常严格的多层次、多步骤的学习，并经过严格的考试和临床应用培养的过程，且这个过程是被严格规范管理的。

放射科医师在有独立执业资格前，首先必须进入医学院学习，毕业后需要通过放射科住院医师的培训。这其中每一阶段都有很多要求和限制，以确保掌握学习和培训的内容，获得相应的基础知识和技术技能，为晋级打下基础。从高中毕业到成为放射科医师，整个过程至少13年。放射科医师在美国是一个备受尊敬、个人职业满意度高、收入高的职业。因此，美国很多放射学专业的学生都愿意通过努力学习和工作来达到其严格的标准。

一、本科

与中国相同。美国学生高中毕业后，可申请进入大学接受教育。大学本科教育一般为4年，但是医学院例外，需要4年本科学习后方能申请医学院。每所医学院对于入校的学生都有其独特的要求，学生都必须经过1年的基础课学习，包括生物学、普通化学、有机化学和物理。学校也鼓励学生学习数学、英语和生物化学。有些本科院校开设了医科预科专业，以帮助学生掌握一些医学技能，为以后进入医学院做准备。但大多数学生同时也可以学习自己感兴趣的其他领域的课程。有些医学院更希望学生学习非传统领域的知识。对医学感兴趣的学生可以花时间在医疗机构工作，做志愿者，或参加研究以获得经验，同时展示自己对医学的强烈的兴趣。大学学业完成后，学生们获得理学学士或文学学士学位。大学期间没有达到医学预科标准的学生可以选择相关的学士后课程项目，通过这些课程就有资格申请医学院。

二、医学院

医生是一个非常受尊重和高收入的职业。医学院入学要求很高，而且招收数量有限。绝大多数的申请者来自美国和加拿大。一流医学院的录取率只有5%。由于录取率很低，每个学生平均会申请14所学校。医学院学制4年。虽然有些学校提供学费资助和奖学金，但是学生1年的学费仍在50 000美元左右。

医学院的申请，一般在大学本科快结束时开始。学生必须有教授的推荐信和自己的个人简介。简介包括报考医学院的原因、自己的研究经历、社区服务的经历和医学经验。学生需要参加一个国家级标准化考试，即医学院入学考试（MCAT）。考试的重点是生物学、物理学、语言推理和写作技巧。学生向感兴趣的学校递交申请，并接受评估。评估项目包括本科的学习成绩、本科院校的声誉、MCAT的分数、推荐信、志愿者活动、研究经历、医学经验、发表过的学术文章等。如果达到基本标准，接下来将会参加一个面试。在面试的过程中，申请者将被问及生活经历、对医学的兴趣和申请方面的很多细节。面试通过后，学校就会发出录取通知。

医学院的课程包括临床前期和临床期两部分。传统的模式为入学后前2年（临床前期）是课堂教育，第1年主要学习生物化学、解剖学、生理学、免疫学和流行病学；第2年，将增加临床病理学和临床医学概论。第3、4年是临床期的学习，学生开始在医院和门诊轮转。这一阶段的学生已成为初级临床成员，并体验作为毕业医学生的临床工作和责任。一般需要轮转内科、儿科、外科、精神病科、产科和妇科。此外，允许学生在规定的时间里轮转一些自选科室，如放射诊断科、放射肿瘤科、皮肤科、急诊科等。这可以帮助学生获得完整的教育经历并体验不同专业，有利于他们以后专科的选择。

美国的医学生必须参加两个国家级的标准化考试，即美国医师执照考试（USMLE）的 Step 1 和 Step 2。这个考试主要测试学生对基础学科和临床知识的掌握情况。其他的一些考试由各医学院自行决定。学校还鼓励学生在轮转期间做一些医学研究和临床工作，这样有利于帮助他们将来选择适合自己的专业。医学院毕业后，学生被授予医学博士学位（MD）。在医学院学习期间，学生还可以另花时间攻读医学公共卫生（MPH）、商业（MBA）和法律（JD）的课程。

三、医学院毕业后的培训

医学院毕业后，对有志成为放射诊断医师的学生，必须申请参加放射诊断住院医师培训。

放射诊断学是一个非常理想的专业，因为其收入高、工作时间可以自己掌控、能接触最先进的技术。因此，放射诊断学住院医师培训是竞争最激烈的培训项目之一。需要综合考虑申请者的 USMLE 分数、医学院成绩、推荐信、获得的荣誉、申请报告、发表文章和面试表现。放射诊断学一直是美国医疗竞争最激烈的前 5 名专业之一。排名靠前的专业还包括皮肤学、放射肿瘤学以及外科的一些专科。放射诊断学住院医师培训的申请，一般在医学院的第 4 年开始，申请者需提交教授的推荐信、USMLE 分数和自己的简介。简介包括描述其参加放射诊断住院医师培训的理由、参与的研究和志愿者的经历等。申请合格的将进入面试。面试时会被问及自己参加放射学住院医师培训的目的、申请材料的细节问题和相关的研究及临床学习经历。

住院医师申请者与住院医师培训计划配对的过程被称为"match"（配对）。在所有面试都结束后，放射住院医师培训项目机构会提供 1 份申请者的成绩排名，学生们也会按照自己的考虑对不同机构的住院医师培训项目进行排名。这 2 份表格将分别被提交到一个中央电脑数据库。然后电脑会比较申请者和所有培训项目机构的排名并进行匹配（match）。电脑在计算配对时会优先考虑申请者的要求。例如，申请者优先考虑项目 A，那么电脑会检查项目 A 是否也优先考虑该申请者。如果是，该申请者和培训项目 A 将配对成功。如果不是，电脑会考虑该申请者的第 2 个培训项目，直到所有的项目和申请者的志愿都匹配完毕。培训项目机构和申请者一般会在 3 月底获得配对结果。按法律规定培训项目机构和申请者都必须接受配对的结果。

医学院学生毕业后，大多数医师在从事放射科专业工作时都遵循传统的"1+4+1"的培养模式。第 1 年的基础临床培训，住院医师可以选择内科、儿科或普通外科的临床培训。这 1 年是为后来的放射科亚专业培训提供必要的临床基础。随后是 4 年的放射科住院医师培训和 1 年的放射学亚专业的"fellowship"培训。住院医师通常超时工作，但已经开始有工资收入，年薪 4 万~5 万美元。

放射学住院医师在 4 年的培训期间，需要轮转放射科的核心亚专科，包括全身各系统的放射影像和磁共振成像检查、核医学、超声、乳房影像检查、神经放射科、介入放射科和儿科。轮转的时间通常是以月为单位，在不同的培训项目机构中标准都是统一的。全国范围内，有最短时间限制的培训有核医学（至少 4 个月，包括至少 80 小时的课堂和实验室教学），以及乳房影像检查（至少 12 周，2 年培训时间中最少读写 240 个乳房影像病例）。

住院医师的学习方式一般是听课，上级医师指导下的见习、实习和自学。培训方案有一个全面的教学总纲，旨在提供一个全面的关于放射学的概述。课堂授课通常每天 1~2 小时，一般由放射学教授授课。病例讨论是教学讲座的补充。在病例讨论会上，由带教医师提供一个病例，住院医师首先要描述病例类型，然后列出阳性和阴性的发现，最后给出诊断结果和处理方案。这种模式设计强调制定一个标准化的方案，可以用来评估住院医师独立工作的能力。住院医师还接受放射物理、放射防护、图像处理、放射病理学、分子成像原理、职业精神和职业道德等方面的指导。

在工作日，住院医师通常是第一个研究检查结果的（第一个读片者），当他们写完规定数量的初步读片报告后，放射科主治医师就会定期带领住院医师进行读片和报告书写，这一过程被称为"read out"（读片）。主治医师带教住院医师讨论这些病例的同时，也提供了非正式的教学。经过集体讨论后，会生成 1 份最终报告并提交给相关专科医师。

在第 1 年，住院医师通常不可以独立出具报告，必须在一名更高资历的放射医师指导下工作。在随后的几年中，住院医师逐渐被给予越来越多的责任，工作会越来越独立并开始值夜班，此阶段称为"call"，也即是 24 小时随叫随到。在这一阶段，住院医师独立工作并写出初步报告，如有需要，可以咨询和得到主治医师的帮助。第 2 天，这些初步的报告会由一名主治医师审核并生成最终报告。对于所有住院医师而言，他们出具的读片报告，最终必须由主治医师来审查确认后才完成。带教医师需定期对住院医师进行专业指导。

所有的医疗培训计划，包括放射诊断学，都必须由"研究生医学教育认可委员会"（ACGME）来审核并认可。该委员会确保全国范围内医疗培训项目的标准化，规定并监测住院医师的工作时间、处理有关不公平待遇的投诉，以确保住院医师得到标准的培训。住院医师的工作时间被限制在每周 80 小时（相当于中国的住院总，24 小时随叫随到），平均每周休息 1 天。为了确保该规则和项目计划的顺利执行，ACGME 会定期进行现场审查。如果有某些培训计划不遵守该规则，将会取消其培训资格。住院医师被要求记录一些日常的工作程序汇报给 ACGME，以保证他们得到足够的医学培训课程。

住院医师培训期间，还需完成 1 份关于改进工作质量的方案和 1 项学术研究课题。改进工作质量方案的内容涉及患者防护的改善，提高工作效率或者是提升放射学教育质量。学术研究课题往往采取实验室或临床研究的形式。有的住院医师培训项目提供了专门的研究时间或研究途径，这些项目通常是和一名教授合作，借此帮助发现住院医师自己感兴趣的放射学亚专业。对于以后希望从事理论放射学的学生，要求就他们从事的研究书写论文并发表在学术期刊上。

美国放射学医师认可证书由"美国放射委员会"（ABR）发放，该委员会也是制定培训要求并组织强制性考试的机构。这类考试在住院医师期间被分为 3 部分。物理考试部分为笔试，在培训的第 2 年进行，重点考核应用放射物理学。在培训的第 3 年，读片和写临床报告以书面考试的形式来进行。在培训的最后 1 年，将以口头考试来测试被培训者在这几年所学的全部知识。住院医师的考核完成并通过后，可以独立的工作。

　　许多放射科医师在完成住院医师培训后选择参加进一步的放射专科培训，被称为"fellowship"（类似中国的进修医师）。Fellowship是获得大学医院职位中必不可少的，对获得私人诊所的工作也很有帮助。这需要1年的时间完成，重点是放射学的1个亚专业，这个亚专业是培训者自己选定的。Fellowship的培训没有住院医师培训那么严格和复杂，多数也不会被ACGME认证。多数的fellowship在大学的医学中心。那里有很多优势，比如在某放射亚专科有训练有素的医务人员，并有很多临床案例。Fellowship的收入比住院医师期间稍高点，但一旦完成培训，他们就可以得到更高的工资。Fellowship占据了一个独特的位置，他们是有放射科医师认可证书的医师，但是仍在接受培训。因此，在此段培训期内，他们的作用和住院医师是相似的，他们写的报告还是要经过主治医师审核确认后才最终生效。然而在放射科的其他亚专业，他们却和主治医师很相似，可以独立完成报告。

　　经过正规培训，执业放射医师还需定期接受教育和测试，以保持其职业证书的有效，这一系列过程称"证书维持"（M0C）。放射学医师每年都必须获得一定的"继续医学教育"（CME）学分。学分可以通过参加学术会议、部门病例讨论会、评阅文章、教育培训或致力于继续医学教育教学研讨会。放射学医师每年还必须网上在线进行自我评估测试（SAM），测试主要内容是放射学总论和放射亚专业。每隔10年，放射学医师必须参加专业技能认证的考试，该考试是在计算机上完成的，检测考试者的非解说技能和临床知识。传统上，放射学医师不需参加这样严格的考试。但为了使放射医学专业像其他医学专科一样，这些要求也正慢慢地开始应用于放射学医师。

　　总之，成为执业的放射科医师约需要10余年的学习和培训，期间要求和测试很多。然而，这个过程竞争又非常激烈，不能满足要求的申请者在任何一个环节都有可能被淘汰。放射诊断医师的教育培训是有组织的、非常严谨复杂的结构体系，它保证了全国范围内的放射学医师都达到了较高的统一的标准。最终的结果是一个培训有素的放射学医师能满足医疗系统复杂的、不断的变化。该系统已经被证明能培养出优秀的临床放射学医师、尖端的研究者、受世界尊敬的健康政策的倡导者。放射学是医学领域最令人兴奋和值得期待的专业之一，拥有不断的技术革新，以满足越来越高的要求。

第二章 美国放射诊断学住院医师培养和考试体系概况
（An Introduction to American Radiology Resident Training and Examination System）

美国住院医师的培养和考核是一个相对完整的体系，有众多机构参与，共同保证住院医师培训的质量，由此促进了美国整体医疗服务质量的不断提高。了解和借鉴美国住院医师培养的经验，对中国医师队伍的建设和医疗服务水平的提高具有积极的意义。

在美国，成为住院医师通常要先从医学院毕业并获得医学博士学位，而在进入医学院前，必须首先获得普通大学的学士学位，学生可以在大学里选择学习任何非医学专业，但大多数医学院校要求他们选修一些与医学有关的课程，如普通化学、有机化学、生物学、物理学、英语、数学及统计学等。这些课程也有利于他们通过医学院入学考试。

美国医学院的学制是4年，进入医学院后，医学生们才开始接触医学专业课程。通过医学院4年的学习并考试合格毕业后，他们可以直接获得医学博士学位，然后再通过医师执照考试，并经过全国住院医师匹配组织（the national resident matching program）匹配成为住院医生。

一、与住院医师培养有关的机构

通过了解这些机构及其功能，就会对美国住院医师教育体系有一个总体的认识。

（一）美国毕业后医学教育认证委员会（Accreditation Council for Graduate Medical Education, ACGME）

ACGME 是由美国医学专科委员会（American Board of Medical

Specialties)、美国医院协会(American Hospital Association)、美国医学协会(American Medical Association)、美国医学院协会(Association of American Medical Colleges)和医学专业协会理事会(Council of Medical Specialty Societies)组成的,它依靠其下属的专家审查委员会制订和改进各种评审标准,并按照这些评审标准对全美国的住院医师培训医院和科室进行认证,以保证住院医师的培训质量,从而进一步达到提高美国医疗水平的目的。它也根据住院医师培养医院和科室的规模及师资队伍情况确定其所能招收的住院医师名额。由于美国联邦医疗保险(Medicare)只对通过ACGME认证的医院和科室支付住院医师培养费用,所以美国住院医师培训医院和科室都非常看重ACGME的认证。

(二)美国的大学医学院附属医院或大型医院

美国住院医师的培养大都是在大学医学院附属医院或大型医院里进行的,这些医院为住院医师培养的主办单位(sponsoring institutions)。这些主办单位的住院医师培养科室(resident program)承担具体的住院医师培养工作。ACGME对住院医师培养主办单位进行指导和审查,而指导和审查住院医师培养科室的工作是由ACGME的住院医师培养审查委员会(Residency Review Committee)来完成的。住院医师培养主办单位和科室应致力于卓越的毕业后医学教育和医疗保健工作,ACGME对主办单位和科室的基本要求包括:①主办医院必须通过医疗组织认证联合委员会(Joint Commission on Accreditation of Healthcare Organizations, JCAHO)或其他公认的认证机构的认可。②必须通过ACGME的初次和定期检查。③必须确保所有住院医师培训科室能够给住院医师提供由ACGME提出的六大技能培训,这六大技能包括医学知识(medical knowledge)、病人治疗护理(patient care)、职业素质(professionalism)、人际交流技能(interpersonal and communication skills)、实践中学习和完善(practice-based learning and improvement)及整体观念行医(systems-based practice)。④必须成立毕业后医学教育委员会(Graduate Medical Education Committee)。住院医师培养主办单位必须成立一个由行政官员、各科室负责住院医生培养的主任、教师、住院医师代表和行政人员组成的毕业后医学教育委员会,该委员会负责住院医师和科室之间的协调工作，包括建立和落实有关住院医师教育质量和工作环境的政策，还负责所有 ACGME 评审文件的管理，查看各科室严格按照 ACGME 要求的住院医生培训计划及对不符合 ACGME 要求的更正计划。委员会要确保每个科室在住院医师的选用、待遇、评估、处罚、晋升及解雇的处理方面符合 ACGME 的要求，还要确保每个科室有合适教程，主办单位和科室不滥用住院医师，在工作时间方面符合 ACGME 关于最长工作时间的规范。毕业后医学教育委员会的一个重要的活动内容是内部审查住院医师培训科室。这一活动由本单位非评审科室的教授、住院医师和与住院医师培训有关的行政人员共同参与，通常在两次 ACGME 评审的中间进行，以便给各科室足够的时间依照 ACGME 的要求对住院医生培训的各个方面进行内部审查，并在下次 ACGME 审查之前改正不符合 ACGME 要求的地方。内部审查时会翻阅有关住院医师培训的书面文件，采访科室成员、教师和住院医师，每次内部审查结束时，该委员会将会出具 1 份评审报告，指出评审科室不符合 ACGME 要求的地方并提出更正建议。⑤能够提供住院医生足够的经济资助以及关于他们雇用、福利、假期和医疗保险的正式书面文件。⑥能够保证住院医师能匿名评价教授和轮转亚科，可以参与和他们的培训及病人诊疗有关委员会和医学生及低年住院医生的教学。

（三）Medicare 和退伍军人事务部 (Department of Veterans Affairs)

在美国，培养住院医师的经费主要由 Medicare 提供。2001 年，Medicare 在这方面的开支是 82 亿美元，其中 26 亿美元直接用于住院医师培养，56 亿美元为非直接培养费用。直接的住院医师培养费主要包括住院医师的教育、工资和福利以及教授的工资，直接住院医师培养费用平均分摊到每个住院医师身上每年是 4 万~12 万美元。在美国，6 年住院医师平均税前工资分别是 4.6 万美元、4.8 万美元、5.0 万美元、5.2 万美元、5.4 万美元和 5.65 万美元。非直接培养费用是 Medicare 用来补偿教学医院的，主要用于支付由于住院医师培养所致病人费用的增加和诊疗效率的下降（如更多的仔细检查项目和更长的住院时间），这些费用并没有包括在 Medicare 的诊断相关组（DRGs）付款系统中。

另外一个大的住院医师培养资助单位是退伍军人事务部（Department of Veterans Affairs），它资助了美国 10% 的住院医师培养。还有其他机构，如美国国防部、美国卫生部和美国州政府等机构，但它们仅资助培养很少一部分住院医师。

（四）各个医学学科的专业学会

各个医学学科的专业学会也参与住院医师的培养。以放射住院医师的培养为例，美国放射学院（The American College of Radiology, ACR）通过每年住院医师的在职考试来评价住院医师的水平及其培养医院和科室的培训效果 ACR 制定各项临床实践指南、技术标准和检查方法的适用标准，已广泛用于放射诊断住院医师的培养。美国放射学委员会（American Board of Radiology, ABR）则通过其放射专科医师认证考试来保证放射科医师的质量。

通过对上述与住院医师培养有关机构的介绍，可以了解到美国住院医师培训体系是比较完善的，各种相关机构从各个方面保证住院医师教育质量。

二、美国住院医师的培养和考试系统（以放射科为例）

（一）美国放射诊断住院医师的培养

美国的放射科住院医师培训时间是 5 年，其中第 1 年是在临床科室进行临床医学的训练，大多数放射科住院医师在这 1 年里会选择内科或者外科。后 4 年是在放射科进行放射诊断学的训练，在这 4 年里，住院医师还需要通过美国放射学委员会的认证考试。在放射科进行的临床训练包括以下几个方面：

1. 进行临床放射亚科轮转

这些亚科包括神经五官放射诊断、心血管放射诊断、胸部放射诊断、乳腺影像诊断、腹部放射诊断、小儿放射诊断、心血管介入放射学、妇科放射诊断、超声波诊断、骨关节放射诊断及核医学。在临床放射亚科的轮转中，他们和主治医师一起讨论应该对病人采用什么检查方案，并就影像学检查所见讨论应该如何诊断和鉴别诊断，并协助临床制订治疗方案。在轮转中，主治医师常常是手把手地教他们，住院医师的临床技能、医学道德和作风大都是在这时候学到的。为了适应 ABR 的新的认证考试（见后文），在放射学培训的最后 1 年，住院医师应能在科室允许范围内选择和参与一些专业的轮转,包括普通放射和他们计划将来从事的专业,为进入临床实践做好准备。

2. 临床教学

即读片教学和课堂教学。临床教学在各个教学医院有所不同,一般来说医学院附属医院的教学活动比较多,而社区医院的临床教学相对要少一些。

(1)读片教学:是在临床剩余时间里由主治医师给住院医师讲病例。

(2)课堂教学:在大多数医院,多是在中午吃饭时由各个亚科的教师轮回讲课,一般是45分钟~1.5小时,课堂教学可以是系统讲课或者病例讨论。

3. 夜晚值班

2年以上的住院医师任全科的夜晚值班,他们在主治医师的指导下,在晚上可以对病人出具临时诊断报告。主治医师在第2天与值夜班的住院医师讨论晚上值班遇到的病例,并出正式诊断报告,及时纠正住院医师临时诊断报告中的错误。

4. 医学物理教学

该课程规划是由美国医学物理师协会(American Association of Physicists in Medicine)和ACGME的住院医师培养审查委员会确定的。每位住院医师必须至少有700小时(约4个月)的临床核医学训练和经验,必修的80小时的课堂和实验室教学,内容涉及放射诊断物理学、辐射生物学、辐射保护、放射仪器工作原理、基本分子成像、放射核素化学及其安全使用和质量控制,以及注入人体内用于诊断和治疗的其他药物的生物学和药理学知识。ABR新的住院医师核心考试将强调医学物理学知识的考核(见后文),医学物理学讲座将是所有住院医师参加的每周定期课程。临床教授将物理问题纳入病例讨论教学中,包括"如何让这个图像质量得到改善呢?什么是某一伪影来源?你会如何设计某个病人的影像检查?如何减少不必要的辐射照射?"这样可以保证住院医师能安全、有效、妥善地使用各种放射学技术为病人服务。

5. 行医技能

同所有住院医师一样,ACGME要求放射住院医师也要具有包括医学知识、病人治疗护理、职业素质、人际交流技能、实践中学习和完善及整体观念行医的六大技能。

（1）医学知识（medical knowledge）：是指医师必须掌握已成定论的和不断发展的生物医学、临床医学、流行病学和社会行为科学方面的知识及其在病人疾病诊疗上的应用。放射科医师应能做到：①熟练掌握医学知识及其在医学影像学中的应用，结合临床给出合理的有临床意义的影像学诊断和鉴别诊断；②能做出适当的临床诊断治疗计划；③了解影像设备的工作原理；④能够使用多种信息资源获取科学数据；⑤掌握科学实验设计和实施原则。

（2）病人治疗护理（patient care）：是指医师必须能够提供病人富有同情心的、适当的、有效的诊断和治疗，以解决病人的健康问题和促进病人的康复。放射科医师应当能够做到：①收集病人必要和准确的病史；②根据临床提出的问题和相关的临床、放射、病理诊断结果，制定合理的诊疗计划，确保正确的检查方法的选用和实施，提出合理的诊断和鉴别诊断以及治疗方案，出具书面诊断报告和口头病例报告；③了解电子病历信息系统；④能使用网络系统进行文献检索，以丰富医学知识；⑤了解各种放射检查的辐射剂量，掌握减少医护人员和病人辐射剂量的方法。

（3）职业素质（professionalism）：是指医师必须具有履行专业职责和遵守伦理规范的素质，放射科医师和其他医师一样应具有：①利他主义精神，即把病人和他人的利益放在自身利益之上；②同情心，即应理解和尊重病人及其家庭和其他医护人员；③卓越性，即对病人高度负责，在职业生涯做到活到老学到老；④诚实心，即以诚相待病人和医护人员；⑤正确处理利益冲突，即能妥善处理病人、厂商等各个方面的关系，避免利益冲突；⑥正确处理人际关系，即不因为宗教、种族、性别或教育的差异歧视他人，不进行性或其他类型的骚扰；⑦举报不称职医师，了解不称职医师的含义及防范。由于身体、精神、滥用酒和毒品等原因造成的不称职医师会对病人的诊疗造成损害，有义务举报这种医生；⑧积极的工作习惯，包括准时和专业精神；⑨理解生物医学伦理学原则；⑩坚持保密原则，不泄露病人信息；⑪理解用人体作为研究对象的伦理学问题。

（4）人际交流技能（interpersonal and communication skills）：是指医师必须掌握人际交流技能，以便有效地与病人、家属及医疗卫生专业人员进行信息交流和协作。放射科医师应能做到：①提供明确的书面影像报告，包括合理的诊断、鉴别诊断以及进一步检查和复查的建议；②如有紧急或意外影像学发现（如肺栓塞和夹层动脉瘤等），应及时直接告诉医生或合适的临床人员，并且在报告中写明；③面对面或打电话与医生、病人及其家属和技术支持人员交流；④有和病人谈话获得病人知情同意书（informed consent）的能力，包括向病人解释手术操作或治疗方法的目的、好处、其他可能的疗法及可能出现的并发症。

（5）实践中学习和完善（practice-based learning and improvement）：是指医师在医学实践中有能力进行自我评价、评估和合理采用科学证据、终身学习以便不断改善临床工作。放射科医师和其他医师一样应能做到：①总结实践经验，不断地提高观察、认知、综合、分析影像的能力和操作技能；②正确严格地应用科学文献；③了解循证医学（evidence-based medicine）及其在临床实践中的应用；④使用多种信息资源终身学习，以便不断改善诊疗护理的水平；⑤鼓励他人，包括学生、同行和其他卫生保健专业人员学习。

（6）整体观念行医（systems-based practice）：是指住院医师应当知道整体保健系统，并能在此系统中从事医疗实践，能有效地调用该系统中其他资源，以便提供最佳的医疗保健。放射科医师和其他医师一样应当做到：①能设计具有低成本高效益的诊疗计划；②了解医疗保健的资金来源，包括 Medicare，美国补助医疗保险（Medicaid）、退伍军人事务部、国防部、公共卫生系统、雇主提供的私人保健计划和病人的个人资金；③知道基本的医疗收费方法；④知道国家的医疗管理系统，包括各州的行医执照发行权威机构、国家和地方公共卫生法规和监管机构、Medicare 和 Medicaid 以及医疗组织认证联合委员会；⑤了解临床行政管理原则，如预算、病例和各种记录保存，以及职员招募、雇用、监督和管理。

（二）放射诊断住院医师考核方法

1. 传统 ABR 认证考试

ABR 传统的认证考试分为 2 次笔试和 1 次口试，分别在培训的不同年限进行。2 次笔试分别在住院医师培训的第 2~4 年进行，第 2、3 年放射住院医师笔试考的是放射物理学，第 3、4 年住院医师的笔试内容是临床放射学。第5年放射住院医师考临床放射学口试。放射物理学笔试的内容是放射科的基础知识，包括放射物理、放射药物剂量学等等；临床放射学笔试的内容是放射科的临床知识。2次笔试的形式都是多项选择题。

口试在第5年结束时进行，口试是ABR认证考试中难度最大的一项，形式是多站病例考试，共有11站，包括胸部放射诊断、腹部放射诊断、神经五官放射诊断、泌尿放射诊断、介入放射诊断、小儿放射诊断、乳腺影像诊断、妇科放射诊断等内容，也包括1站超声、1站核医学，1站虚拟心脏放射学。之所以叫虚拟心脏放射是因为这一考试不是单独进行的，而是在胸部放射诊断、介入放射学、小儿放射诊断和核医学站中进行。最后考官们把所有心脏放射病例从这几站中挑出来单独计分，作为心脏放射学亚科的成绩。

2. 放射诊断ABR认证考试

（1）核心考试（core exam）：2013年开始使用这一考试方法。放射住院医师在放射科训练满36个月后（也就是在他们完成第4年住院医师训练后）方可参加这一核心考试。

该考试是计算机考试，有很多片子，在当地考试中心进行，考试时间为2天。考试将测试解剖、病理、放射诊断学和医学物理学的知识。考生必须通过放射科所有的11个亚科（包括胸部放射诊断、腹部放射诊断、神经五官放射诊断、泌尿放射诊断、介入放射学、小儿放射诊断、乳腺影像诊断、妇产放射诊断、超声诊断学、核医学、心脏放射学）和放射物理才算合格。放射物理学将被整合在试题中，但分开作为一个项目进行评分。所以总共12个项目。

如果有3个或者3个以下项目没有通过叫条件通过。考生可以仅仅补考上次未通过的项目。4个或4个以上项目没有通过为考试失败。失败的考生应重新考所有项目。

（2）认证考试（certifying exam）：2015年开始进行的考试。放射住院医师在完成放射诊断住院医师训练15个月后才有资格参加这一考试。

认证考试也是计算机考试，考试的内容主要是阅读大量的片子，也在当地考试中心进行。有两种认证方式。如果考生想当一名普通放射医师，他就得考放射科所有的11个亚科，即11个模块。如果考生想当一名专业放射医师，需考 5 个模块。其中 3 个模块由考生基于自己的培训、经验和计划在将来从事的专业选择。这 3 个模块的考试比普通放射医师的相应亚科考试要深。其他 2 个模块由 ABR 设计。其中一个 ABR 模块的内容是非诊断技能，如辐射安全、造影剂反应的识别和治疗、错误防范、人际交流能力、敬业精神、职业道德等。另一个 ABR 设计的模块是放射诊断基础知识，例如如何识别被虐待儿童、气胸、休克肠、硬膜下血肿等等。

（3）再次认证考试（maintenance of certification exam）：初次认证考试后每 10 年，每位放射医师需要通过 ABR 主办的和上述专业放射医师的认证考试相当的以及与他们所从事的放射专业有关的考试（practice-profile diagnostic radiology exam），达到再次认证。这一考试即是再次认证考试。

3. ACR 在职考试

这一考试是在每年的 2 月份进行，全美国的放射诊断住院医师在同一时间参加考试。这一考试能使住院医师和全国的同行比较了解他们的学习情况，考试形式是多项选择题，考试的内容是放射物理和临床知识。这一考试也能使培训科室了解他们培养的住院医师水平，以便改善不足之处。

4. 其他考试方法

（1）360°评价工具（360 degree evaluation）：主要用于主观评价住院医师的人际交流技能和职业素质，如遵守专业规则、准时上下班等。这种住院医师评价将由各层次人员进行，如全体教员、护士、技术员、培训科室的协调员、同事、病人及其家属。

（2）放射亚科轮转后评价（end of rotation evaluation）：用于评价住院医师各方面的能力，包括评价住院医师诊断报告质量、口头交流能力，以及行医的安全性等。其优点是快速、容易，缺点是对能力的评价往往过于主观。由于教师往往比较宽容，这项评价更多为总结性评价（summative evaluation）和形成性评价（formative evaluation）。

（3）学习成绩和培养记录（portfolio）：包括①测验分数，参加会议/课程记录；②病例记录和手术备案；③遵守核医学及乳腺影像的培养要求；④遵守学院和科室规则；⑤放射报告评价；⑥自我评估和自我学习计划；⑦参加多学科会议和涉及系统问题解决方案的学习活动记录等。

这一考察方法能用于所有六大能力的评价，可用于形成性和总结性评价，应鼓励学生参与此项活动，否则可能会被取消或忽视。这种考察方法的缺点是费时，需要评价的指标和数据过多，均会影响评价的效率和效果。

（4）临时诊断结果的误差率：在芝加哥大学医院里，晚间值班住院医师读过的片子在第2天由主治医师在医学影像存档与通信系统（picture archiving & communication system, PACS）上出正式报告并且评价住院医师所出的临时报告。共有3种符合情况，即符合、轻微不符合和严重不符合。PACS自动统计每个住院医师的临时诊断结果的误差率。PACS也通过电子邮件告知住院医师临时报告符合情况以及不符合的地方，以便住院医师学习。

（5）临床技能考试：例如，介入放射操作、胃肠道造影术和关节造影术的考察，病人安全和辐射计量问题考察（如记录影像引导操作过程的透视时间），考察治疗模拟造影剂反应（如低血压休克）和预防性给药等。

（6）放射亚科轮换前后考试：这种考试的形式多样，可以是口试、笔试、病例或者多选题。

（7）晚间值班就职前资格认可考试：同放射亚科轮换前后考试一样，这种考试可以采取口试、笔试、病例或者多选题的形式。

（8）本院主办的临床放射学模拟口试：这种考试是为了帮助住院医师通过目前的ABR认证考试而进行的。

（三）放射科住院医师教育培训

下面以美国宾州州立大学医学中心为例介绍目前的美国放射科住院医师教育培训情况。

宾夕法尼亚州立大学建于1855年，位于宾夕法尼亚州的斯泰特科利奇，在全国共有24个分校，现有在校学生80 000多人，共有160多个专业可以授予学士学位，150多个专业可以授予硕士或/和博士学位。设于Hershey的医学中心集教学、科研和医疗服务于一体，为美国乃至全世界培养了大批优秀人才，是一所享有较高声誉的综合性公立医学中心。

1. 培训按系统全面轮转

按照美国医学教育认证委员会（ACGME）规定，放射科住院医师要进行为期5年的培训，第1年进行临床轮转，包括内科、外科、妇产科、儿科、神经科、急诊科等；第2~5年进行专科轮转，包括放射物理学、放射生物学，以及腹部、乳腺、心胸、骨肌、神经、核医学、儿科放射学、腹部和血管超声、血管介入放射学9个亚专业。美国放射学委员会（ABR）规定，在住院医师培训的第4年进行笔试，第5年完成后进行最终的认证考试。宾州州立大学医学中心放射科现有5台磁共振（Siemens 1.5 T 2台、Siemens 3.0T 1台、Philips 3.0T 1台、Bruker 7T 1台）、6台CT（Siemens 16层1台、40层2台、64层2台、128层1台）、1台PET-CT、1台SPECT-CT。每位放射科医生配备4台电脑，2台用于阅片，1台用于写诊断报告，1台用于查阅临床信息及文献。全院实现信息网络共享，放射科医生可以很方便地调阅临床住院患者病历信息和病理信息。医学中心的放射科按系统对专业精细划分，涵盖上述所有亚专业，每个系统都设有相对独立的办公室。该院放射科住院医师共28名，都是从全国各地的申请者中通过面试严格挑选出来的，所有住院医师都要在5年内按计划完成所有系统轮转，每个系统的轮转都对住院医师提出具体的要求和明确的目标。包括：影像检查的操作程序及主要疾病的影像诊断。以腹部放射为例，要熟悉X线平片、胃肠造影、CT和磁共振的检查方法及其原理，掌握常见腹部疾病的诊断（包括腹部外伤、炎症、胃肠道肿瘤、肝胆胰脾以及盆腔病变等），每个系统出组时都要经过严格的考核。因此，医学中心的住院医师工作都非常认真，有着很高的学习热情及学习主动性，遇到问题，都会马上查阅文献、互相讨论、询问教师，对自己书写的报告也是反复推敲，直到满意为止；同时还会积极追踪病理结果，使诊断得到及时反馈。

2. 教学方式多样，注重思维训练

宾州州立大学医学中心放射科每个专业组都由几名资深的主治医师组成，并设有组长，通过多种形式对住院医师进行培训。放射科每天早晨7:30~8:30读片，各专业组都会有各自的病例讨论活动，一般分成2段。前30分钟为教学读片，由一名资深主治医师主持，将准备好的病例展示出来，针对影像检查序列、影像特点、解剖及临床相关的知识，对不同年资的住院医师进行提问。教师一般不直接给出答案，而是引导学生各抒己见，最后再点评。后30分钟一般为疑难病例讨论，针对临床遇到的实际诊断问题，几名主治医师会积极发言，而学生也可以随时提问，气氛十分活跃。平时工作中，住院医师一般通过语音输入影像报告，对每一个病例的征象进行分析。如果遇到疑难问题，每位医师配有专用电脑，存储有丰富的影像学资料，针对各种疾病的特异性影像征象都有详细的图片、解剖及文字说明，可以查阅学习，非常快捷方便。在轮转过程中一般低年住院医师与高年住院医师搭配转组，所有影像报告的诊断最终由一名带教主治医师负责签发。其在复核报告时会对征象进行仔细讲解，深入分析其发生机制，并引导住院医师提出多种不同的可能性，从而进行鉴别诊断。此外，每周一到周五的中午 11:30~13:00 都有住院医师培训课程，按不同系统安排课程表。由一名主治医师通过幻灯片就 1 个专题进行讲解，年轻住院医师按不同年资坐成几排，边听课边进餐。讲课为互动式，可随时提问，主讲教师有时也会组织一些影像病例，每个住院医师都要发言，进行分析和阐述自己的诊断及依据，最后由主讲教师总结。此外，放射科住院医师还需要就自己的专业学习定期进行总结汇报，其表现将记入学习培训评价表。通过不同方式从不同角度训练学生的能力，对住院医师严格要求，注重理论学习，思维方式的训练和实践，长此以往，必将建立缜密的临床思维方式，培养出思维敏捷的医生。

3. 多学科合作，科研氛围浓厚

科研培训是放射科医生培养中的重要组成部分，通过从事科学研究工作，有助于培养客观严谨的科学态度，细致和有条不紊的工作作风。医学中心设有相对独立的磁共振研究所，其综合了临床医学、理工科、生物医学、动物实验以及数据分析等各方面的人才，是真正的多学科人才汇聚的地方。磁共振研究所在嗅觉成像领域处于国际前沿，在嗅觉、味觉等刺激诱导的脑功能成像技术及其临床应用方面独辟蹊径，其研发的嗅觉刺激仪设计严谨，并在应用中不断改进，为嗅觉成像提供了独特的方法。目前他们已与临床神经内科合作，将嗅觉成像分析应用在帕金森病、老年痴呆等领域，并取得了多项科研成果。宾州州立大学医学中心作为美国综合性医院，要求住院医师必须具备较强的科研意识和科研能力，住院医师都会根据自己的兴趣参加 1~2 项科学研究项目，抽出一定时间进行科研工作。研究所每周安排 2 次学术讨论会，由研究所主任主持，大家轮流找到有价值、感兴趣的文献，做成幻灯片，进行学术讨论，分析文章的思路和内容。讲解过程中，大家可以随时打断提问，通过热烈的讨论训练了学生的能力，追踪了研究的最新进展，锻炼了表达能力，有助于挖掘到有价值的科研思路。

第三章　美国超声医学教育模式特点
（Characteristics of the Educational Mode of Medical Ultrasonography in the United State）

超声医学目前已是临床最常用的影像学诊断方法之一。我国超声专业医师的培养模式、规模也经过几代人的努力而日益完善及壮大，已形成本科（临床医疗/医学影像专业）—硕士研究生—博士研究生规范化教育体制，为各级医疗单位培养了大量超声专业医师，促进了医疗水平的整体提高。但不同医疗单位间诊断水平参差不齐，整体与发达国家仍有差距。美国的超声事业起步较早，经过几十年的发展，已形成体制健全、机制成熟、高水平的人才培养模式。笔者曾在美国2所医学院（Oregon Health and Science University, OHSU; Baylor College of Medicine, BCM）及其附属医院从事2年超声影像医学诊断学习，有机会近距离接触美国超声专业人员的培训制度，对其申请、选拔、临床训练、考试与考核方法以及专业证书准入制度等有较深的了解。

一、超声专业工作模式特点

在美国各级医疗机构中，超声专业人员由2部分组成：临床医师和技师，二者分工不同，互相配合完成全部超声诊断工作。一般由技师直接对患者进行超声检查操作，技师不负责诊断，只需要完成病例的全套标准化切面图像采集，并上传至超声影像工作站。具体的图像分析、诊断工作则由各科专科医师完成，一般不设立专门的超声科室。技师并不要求医学专业背景，通过超声专业课程培训及全国统一的超声技术考核（分类详细，腹部、妇产科、小器官等科目需分别考试）后，在上级医师或其他技师指导下完成一定数量的病例操作，即获得相应资质，可受聘于各级医院影像科室担任工作。心血管超声诊断一般由心内科医师进行，腹部超声诊断由放射科医师进行，只有妇产科超声例外，多数由妇产科医师自行操作、诊断。

由于标准化切面的应用，该工作模式对技师来说易于学习掌握，任何一名诊断医师拿到资料后都可以分析图像，独立诊断。另外，由于负责诊断的是临床专科医师，具有强大的专业知识背景，相比仅从事超声医学的超声医师，具有一定的优势。不足之处在于这种模式不利于发挥操作者的主动性，技师不必详细问诊和对病程进行思考，医师却只能依赖技师取得的图像资料进行诊断。如果技师有漏诊，那么医师则不可避免的也发生漏诊。特别在腹部和浅表器官等疾病，由于病灶位置不同，常出现非标准切面，需要操作者灵活掌握。

在我国，多数医院有独立的超声科或B超室，有资质的医师或技师自己操作，并完成诊断。这种模式的优势在于病例采集与诊断之间没有脱节，医师亲自操作，可以边诊断边问诊，获取信息迅速，能及时调整思路，特别是对腹部疾病患者，常常可有意外的发现，最后的诊断往往与申请单上的最初判断有差别。另外，该模式效率高，短期内可完成大量工作，适合我国国情。不足之处在于，虽然医／技师各种疾病的超声诊断都熟悉，专业知识背景面比较广，但就某一类疾病（比如心血管疾病）的了解深度（包括病程、转归和预后）常逊于临床专业医师。

二、医师培养模式特点

在美国，从事超声诊断的临床专科医师的培训，同其他专科医师并无不同，毕业后都要参加住院医师培训。美国的住院医师培训制度是毕业后医学教育的一个重要组成部分，所有医学毕业生都要进行3~5年的住院医师培训教育。以超声影像诊断为例，要熟悉超声成像的方法及其原理、检查程序；掌握各系统（包括消化系、泌尿生殖系等）常见病的标准切面、超声表现、超声造影灌注特点等。各个系统轮转结束后都有相应的考核，因此保证了住院医师的临床水平，为兼任临床影像诊断打下坚实基础。经过严格住院医师培训后，一般都能胜任主治医师的工作，并且具备一定的教学和科研能力。

三、美国超声专业教学形式特点

超声是一门实践性极强的学科，临床知识与操作手法缺一不可，因此教学也必须和实践紧密结合，才会取得较好效果。就笔者的自身感受，美国的超声专业教学主要有以下特点：

（一）重视师资力量

在美国，常常以大学的系为单位，整个大学、多家医院的许多高水平主治医师组成一个整体的教师队伍，通过多种形式的教学对住院医师实行联合培养，使刚毕业的住院医师有更多的接触各种病例和学习的机会。平时一名主治医师指导一名住院医师，共同阅读分析超声图像，先由住院医师对正常、异常征象进行逐一描述，然后主治医师进行复核，对征象和诊断进行讲解，并修正诊断结果。

（二）教学方式多种多样

许多教学医院每天中午在固定的报告厅设有针对不同年资住院医师的讲座，时间为1小时，由主治医师主讲。讲课是互动式，气氛轻松（住院医师的午饭时间，可边听边吃），可随时提问讨论。每天还有各专科举行的专题讲座，主要是针对Fellow（相当于前主治），住院医师也可参加。另外每天还有各专科的病例讨论会，有2种形式：一种是主治医师主持，拿出疑难病例，让Fellow读，然后由主治医师主讲；还有一种是Fellow主持，由Fellow轮流准备，将1周内有意义的病例做成幻灯片来讨论，其他的Fellow发言，然后由主持的Fellow介绍相关临床知识和影像表现及鉴别诊断，整个过程中由一名教授负责修正错误意见。笔者所在的德州儿童医院（Texas Children's Hospital, TCH）心脏科，在培训心脏科医师时，针对讲解先天性心脏病的超声诊断课程，每周安排1次病理课，病理科医师并不以讲解为主，而是带来各种各样、各年龄阶段的先心病心脏大体标本，列出不同诊断，由学生仔细观察、选择答案，可自行讨论、随时提问。这种课程使学生印象深刻，胜于任何语言讲解，笔者虽从事超声诊断多年，但是每当看到复杂先心病的标本，常感到真正的异常解剖与平时仅凭超声切面在脑海中建立的空间结构仍有不同。通过多形式的教学模式，不仅提高了住院医师的理论知识，也增加了接触各种病例的机会，提高了对相关疾病影像的诊断分析水平。

（三）广泛开展兴趣性研究

在完成临床工作之余，住院医师会有机会根据自己的兴趣选择一些项目参加科学研究。知名度较大的一些研究型医院，每年的科研经费可达到医院总支出的1/4。TCH 的医师多数在知名的贝勒医学院（Baylor College of Medicine, BCM）任职，BCM 作为全美较大的研究型医院，要求住院医师必须培养较强的科研意识和科研能力。住院医师可自愿参加研究项目，抽出一定时间进行科研工作、撰写和发表科研文章。Fellow 则要求必须有独立完成的科研项目，作为结业时考核是否合格的标准之一。多数科室会安排杂志俱乐部（Journal Club）进行学术讨论学习，由一名住院总或科秘书负责安排，大家轮流找有价值、感兴趣的文章学习讨论，分析文章的具体内容，不仅有利于了解当前的研究动态，而且有助于提高科研水平。讨论的内容十分广泛，不仅仅限于科学性研究，还涉及医学伦理学、科研道德和方法等等，不一而足，形式不拘一格，学术气氛浓厚而且十分自由。在笔者曾参加过的一次 Journal Club 中，一位教授就以发表在著名杂志 Circulation 上的一篇文章为例，逐步分析该文章在研究方法和写作上的疏漏，有理有据，环环相扣，最后总结怎样设计临床实验，写好科研文章，给学生以很大启发。

第四章　意大利影像医学教学与临床模式特点
（Characteristics of Teaching and Clinical Model of Medical Imaging in Italy）

随着医学影像仪器的快速发展，医学影像学已经成为临床最重要的辅助诊断方式之一，影像医学教学也已成为临床专业教学的重要组成部分。本文研究者在意大利罗马生物医学大学（Universita Campus Bio-medico di Roma，CBM）医院影像科进行培训学习期间，近距离地接触和了解了意大利的影像医学教学和临床情况，通过总结其专业特点及差异，对我国医学影像学教学与临床水平的提升是很好的借鉴。

一、影像医学教学

（一）培养模式与课程设置

意大利高校的医学专业均开设于综合性大学的医学院，如罗马大学、帕多瓦大学、米兰大学等。医学院招收高中毕业生，入学有名额限制，并要通过严格的专业考试。学制与教学模式执行欧盟标准即博洛尼亚协议，本科3年、硕士2年、博士根据不同专业一般为3~5年。临床医学专业为六年制，毕业后颁发硕士学位，影像技术为三年制本科，毕业后颁发学士学位。

与我国传统的前3~4年理论学习，后1~2年临床见习实习的医学院课程设置不同，意大利医学院每一学年均设置医学基础理论课、人文实践活动和临床实习，使学生能够理论与实践相结合。以CBM大学三年制影像与放疗技术专业为例，第1学期9~11月上课，之后进入相应的临床影像科室实习3个月，第2年2月左右进行期末考试。其他大学的课程设置与CBM大学基本相同，只是不同专业、不同学年的实习时间略有不同。有些专业可灵活安排临床科室的实习时间，但每年必须取得一定的实践学分。除临床见习实习外，学生还必须参加多种实践活动，如社会活动、研讨会、讲座、医患接触等活动，提倡以学生为中心的自主式学习。

意大利医学院没有设立专门培养影像诊断医师的医学影像学本科或硕士研究生专业。影像诊断医师必须经过医学院校临床医学专业学习6年后，进入医院，再进行5年左右影像专科培训，培训考试合格并被医院正式聘用后才能担任。影像技师则是三年制的影像技术专业本科毕业后，通过技师考试取得相应资质聘用上岗。

在影像诊断医师的专科培训过程中，每位学生都配有1位资深的影像医生作为培训导师，按照规定完成放射、CT、磁共振和超声等科室的轮转。专科培训期间主要以实践和自主学习为主，每天需要完成一定数量的影像读片，并写出初步诊断意见。遇到疑难病例可以自主上网检索相关文献、查阅病例资料，也可互相讨论或请教导师。科室每天开展1次病例讨论，选取疑难病例，由资深医生主持，大家各抒己见，积极发言，讨论热烈，最后由教师点评。此外，培训期间还要参加各种类型的讲座，优秀的学生

医学影像学专业英语

会被导师安排少量的本科生带教工作。由于 CBM 大学医院的影像科是罗马影像中心，因此科研培训也是专科培训期间的一项任务，要求学生必须掌握基本的科研方法，并有能力承担导师研究的部分工作。

（二）人文教育

意大利医学专业课程设置一般分为专业课、临床相关课程、基础课和人文科学等。在基础与专业课程设置上与国内医学专业相似，但人文课程的比例高于国内同类专业。以培养影像技师的影像技术与放疗专业为例，短短 3 年学习时间，学生需要完成伦理学、护理科学、遗传学、生物伦理学、人类学与医学史、社会心理学、临床心理学等近 10 门人文科学与伦理科学课程，临床医学专业还要在人文科学理论学习的基础上完成社会实践活动。大部分医学院校开设的人文课程国内医学院校鲜有涉及，如生物伦理学、人类学与医学史、社会心理学等。从一名技师的培养过程可以看出，意大利对人文科学教育的重视程度。医务工作者必须具有足够高的人文素养，从接受医学教育开始就应该受到人文主义的熏陶。

（三）继续教育

意大利影像医学的继续教育主要在医院内开展,继续教育的形式多样,主要以定期举办各类讲座和病例讨论会为主,也有外出参加学术会议的机会,但进修培训机会较少。院内的讲座参加人员主要为科室医生,特别是低年资医生和见习实习学生。也有较大规模和较高层次的讲座或论坛、讨论等,参与人员为医院各相关科室医生。继续教育内容广泛,涉及多门学科,不仅有影像方面的新进展、特殊病例讨论等,还邀请病理、核医学、外科等相关科室的医生进行授课。讲座或课后都有讨论,参与者各抒己见,积极发言,不仅提高了医生的理论水平,也增加了临床经验,拓宽了影像诊断的思路。

二、影像医学临床

意大利医院的影像诊断科通常分为常规 X 线、CT、磁共振（MR）、超声、乳腺钼靶和导管室几个部门。影像科技师的岗位一般相对固定，医生为轮班制，轮流在各部门诊断阅片，但每位医生都有自己的专业方向。资深影像医生工作安排相对固定，如介入、冷冻治疗等都有专门的医生操作，但每周也有2天时间到其他部门轮转。轮转促使影像医生熟练掌握各种影像检查和诊断技术，在诊断疾病时能够结合多种检查方式，扬长避短，更好地完成疾病的影像诊断和治疗。如CBM影像科医生在进行超声介入穿刺活检时，首先应用超声仪器实时引导穿刺针到达包块后，然后进行CT腹部扫描，确认穿刺针位置，再在超声引导下实时穿刺活检，拔出穿刺针之后再次进行CT检查，观察有无包块所在脏器出血等并发症。这样的介入活检，将超声与CT完美结合，很好地利用超声多方位实时性和CT的准确性，又同时避免腹部气体和超声声束偏移可能造成的不良影响，高质量地完成了介入任务。

除急诊外的患者均采用预约制，一般的影像检查平均每30分钟预约一位患者。因此影像科医生检查时间充足，影像扫描方式更多。以脊柱磁共振检查为例，CBM医院的影像科采用22种扫描方式，而国内医院由于患者过多，时间所限，一般只采用5~7种。但门诊患者预约时间较长，如MR检查，需等待6个月左右，普通的超声检查也需1~2个月的预约时间。

影像诊断医师在诊断时可调阅系统中患者所有的临床资料和影像检查信息，有更多的时间与患者沟通，可详细询问病史及相关临床症状，并且诊断标准可根据国际标准随时更新，诊断时遇到疑难病例也能及时上网搜寻相关信息。

参考文献

［1］陈维益. 英汉医学辞典 [M]. 2 版. 上海：上海科学技术出版社, 1997.

［2］刘明, 程彦, 韦建辉. 医学英语学习与论文撰写 [M]. 北京：人民卫生出版社, 2019.

［3］Cylys B A, Wedding M E. Medical terminology Systems[M]. 7th ed. New York: F. A. Davis Company, 2012.

［4］Chabner D. The language of medicine[M]. 11th ed. Beijing: Peking University Medical Press, 2017.

［5］Newman W A. Dorland's illustrated medical dictionary[M]. 30th ed. Philadelphia: W. B. Saunders Company, 2003.

［6］Stewart M B, Natalie PB. The human body: Structure and function in health and disease[M]. 2nd ed. St. Louis: The C. V. Mosby Company, 1980.

［7］Austrin M G, Austrin H R. Young's learning medical terminology[M]. 6th ed. St. Louis: The C.V. Mosby Company, 1987.

［8］Barbara A G, Mary Ellen Wedding. Medical terminology: A systems approach[M]. 2nd ed. Philadelphia: F A. Davis Company, 1988.

［9］Anthony L S. Mastering medical language[M]. 3th ed. New Jersey: Prentice-Hall, Inc, Englewood Cliffs, 1982.

［10］Firkin B G, Whitworth J A. Dictionary of medical eponyms [M]. Lancs: The Partheonon Publishing Group Limited, 1989.

［11］Laurie B. English word-formation[M]. Cambridge: Cambridge University Press, 1983.

［12］Quirk R，et al. A comprehensive grammar of the English language [M]. London: Longman，1985.

［13］Laurence U. Suffixes and other word-final elements of English[M]. Detroit: Gale Research Company，1982.

［14］张燕琳，华明清，胥胜江. 医学影像技术专业英语 [M]. 天津：天津科学技术出版社，2019.

［15］Grimm L J, Maxfield C M, 陈君彦. 美国的放射学医师培训 [J]. 中华放射学杂志,2011,45(11):1083-1085.

［16］王志群，苏壮志，杜祥颖，等. 美国宾州州立大学放射科住院医师教育培训启示 [J]. 中华医学教育探索杂志,2014(9):878-880.

［17］郑敏娟，潘峰. 美国超声医学教育模式特点及对我国超声专业教育的启示 [J]. 西北医学教育,2010,18(5):930-933.

［18］段云燕，黄明刚. 意大利影像医学教学和临床模式特点与启示 [J]. 中华医学教育探索杂志,2015(9):881-884.